Quality Matters:
From Clinical Care to Customer Service

Quintessentials of Dental Practice – 31
General Dentistry/Practice Management – 4

Quality Matters:

From Clinical Care to Customer Service

By
Raj Rattan

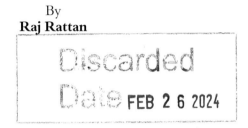
Editor-in-Chief: Nairn H F Wilson
Editor General Dentistry/Practice Management: Raj Rattan

Quintessence Publishing Co. Ltd.
London, Berlin, Chicago, Paris, Milan, Barcelona, Istanbul,
São Paulo, Tokyo, New Delhi, Moscow, Prague, Warsaw

British Library Cataloguing in Publication Data

Rattan, Raj
  Quality matters: from clinical care to customer service. – (Quintessentials of dental practice; v. 31)
    1. Dentistry – Practice 2. Dentist and patient
    I. Title II. Wilson, Nairn H. F.
    617.6

ISBN-13: 9781850971009

ISBN-13: 978-1-85097-100-9

Foreword

One of the primary concerns of patients is quality of care. Today, quality of care, as considered in this most welcome addition to the now substantial *Quintessentials* series, is a broad concept, embracing all aspects of the patient experience. In this carefully crafted book, Dr Rattan aims to help colleagues better understand how to satisfy, and wherever possible exceed, patients' ever increasing expectations of quality of care. The aims and objectives of the book have been surpassed through Dr Rattan's skilful consideration of the relevant theory and his authoritative approach to the necessary attitudes towards quality and quality improvement to optimise the delivery of care in the clinical practice of dentistry. *Quality Matters: From Clinical Care to Customer Service* is an engaging, easy-to-read text, peppered with advice and guidance of immediate practical relevance. Understanding and applying the many interrelated aspects of quality of care should be considered an integral element of professional ethics and professionalism, as viewed in our changing society. As such, *Quality Matters: From Clinical Care to Customer Service* should be essential reading for all those with limited knowledge of quality issues in oral healthcare provision. Moreover, and in common with Dr Rattan's other books in the *Quintessentials* series, this book includes numerous pearls of wisdom for even the most experienced of practitioners. The few hours necessary to read and digest this concise, thought-provoking book, will be time well spent. What good is care that lacks quality?

Nairn Wilson
Editor-in-Chief

This book is for Ella, Alex and Anna

Preface

The challenge of writing this book was a challenge of interpretation.

How should I interpret the term *"quality"*? Narrowly defined, quality refers to clinical outputs – periodontal treatment, crowns and bridges, simple and complex restorations, and so on. A broader interpretation would include the quality of the process of care, the quality of the service, the quality of the people delivering the care, and the quality of the environment in which the care was provided. Each of these facets is in itself an aggregate of smaller components, so how far do we need to explore each individual component?

I have chosen to take the broadest view on quality and thus include elements that I believe to be relevant to general dental practice. There is more to quality than implementing a system or working towards a given standard; it is about an attitude of mind that makes us want to improve the way we work and live. Attitude is the fuel of ambition.

Throughout this book, I have referred to users of our services as *"patients"*. It has become fashionable to talk about *"customers"* and *"clients"* in dentistry, but the use of these terms has been used only where they appear in verbatim citations from other texts. To serve a patient is a privilege bestowed only to healthcare workers; it embraces all the desirable elements important to clients and customers but also includes the unique ethical attributes associated with healthcare.

The reader should be aware of one omission from this text. It relates to an important element of quality and that is risk management and patient safety. This subject has been covered in depth in a previous book in this series, *Risk Management in General Dental Practice*.

Professor John Øvretveit, Director of Research at the Medical Management Centre, Karolinska Institutet, Stockholm, is a respected authority on quality in healthcare. His view that "a quality system is based on underlying theory about what needs to be done to provide a quality service" has influenced the structure of this text. The theory is important – it drives the implementation of quality initiatives in the context of our own working environment.

If we wanted to build a car engine, we would need to know and understand the theory behind the design. We would welcome information on how others have approached engine design and we would ask for guidance on how and where to begin. That is what I have aimed to do in this book.

The value of the theory, ideas and examples is only realised when the rubber hits the road. That remains the driver's responsibility.

Raj Rattan

Acknowledgement

My sincere thanks to all those who willingly and unselfishly gave their permission to quote and reference their work in the preparation of this book. Their responses to my requests for information and advice were always positive and immediate; their individual contributions are cited in the text.

Contents

Chapter 1
Introduction

Aim

The aim of this chapter is to provide an overview of the meaning and inter-pretation of quality in the broadest sense and to highlight some of the key benefits of a commitment to quality.

Outcome

The reader will have an understanding of how the meaning of quality can vary in relation to its context and the relevance of the various interpretations in everyday dental practice.

Introduction

Healthcare quality has been on the agenda of scholars, policy analysts, providers and patients for many decades. By the 1970s, Avedis Donabedian had established his model for assessing quality on the basis of structure, process and outcome. A decade later, patient safety, risk management and appropriateness of care were added to the common list of measurement vari-ables.

Many practice websites, leaflets and marketing materials make references to quality, but few are explicit about its meaning and interpretation.

"Quality … you know what it is, yet you don't know what it is. But that's self-contradictory. But some things are better than others, that is, they have more quality. But when you try to say what the quality is, apart from the things that have it, it all goes poof! There's nothing to talk about ..." So wrote Robert M. Pirsig in his book, *Zen and the Art of Motorcycle Main-tenance* (p.163). In his PhD thesis "On Quality of Dental Care", Poorter-man makes a similar point that: "A person generally is able to make an image of the meaning of that particular word and recognises it when in contact, but it is difficult to give the exclusive right description."

The meaning of quality is explored further in Chapter 2.

In general dental practice, quality is the measure of how good dental health outcomes are, and can be evaluated for at least two components. The technical element of quality care looks at the components of clinically appropriate diagnostic decision-making, treatment planning and execution and any required follow-up.

The personal element includes the degree to which the patient perceives being cared for – confidence, compassion, trust – and an overall sense of satisfaction from the practice as a whole. While the technical element of quality is relatively objective, and the personal relatively subjective, both are measurable.

Writing in the British Dental Journal in 1996, Mindak points out that: "Patients judge the dental service they receive by the interaction with the service providers – the dentist and his or her staff – as they are unable to judge the technical quality of the service."

The interactive and organisational elements make us unique; we may know the recipe for quality in general practice but the way we choose to apply it results in a blend that is unique to each and every practice.

The Dutch National Council for Public Health has developed a framework that describes quality in clinical practice (Fig 1-1).

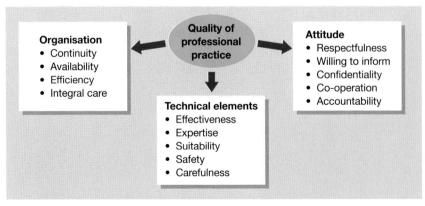

Fig 1-1 The Dutch National Council for Public Health framework for quality in clinical practice.

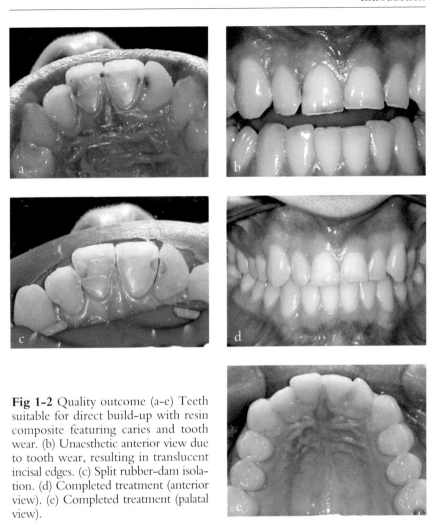

Fig 1-2 Quality outcome (a-e) Teeth suitable for direct build-up with resin composite featuring caries and tooth wear. (b) Unaesthetic anterior view due to tooth wear, resulting in translucent incisal edges. (c) Split rubber-dam isolation. (d) Completed treatment (anterior view). (e) Completed treatment (palatal view).

A quality clinical outcome will result from a combination of the aspects under each of the three domains, some of which will be more important than others for each patient experience (Fig 1-2).

Challenges

We live in the age of the mixed economy and there are challenges in managing quality in this context. Many practices choose to provide care and

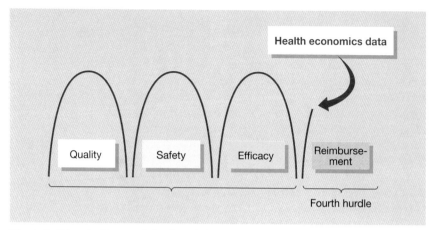

Fig 1-3 The challenge of the fourth hurdle.

services through private and public sector funding. These practices must satisfy the meaning of quality as defined by the stakeholders of all the parties. Who is the customer in the public sector – the commissioner or the patient? Is there shared status? Equity is the priority in many public sector services. The requirement to maintain a balance between the needs of the individual and the needs of the community means that a particular person cannot always have everything. Is it then possible for the provider to satisfy both the patient and the commissioner? A patient who is denied a service because it is not available through the public sector is unlikely to consider the public service in terms of quality, but another patient who is able to access the service at a time of acute need will have the opposite view.

The definition of quality in a public service is based upon the values and expectations of key stakeholders. There is a requirement on the part of the commissioners to deliver value and the need to use public funds in a clinically and cost-effective way. All members of a caring profession would be willing to jump the hurdles of quality, patient safety and clinical efficacy, but not all feel able to accept the funding provided to tackle these challenges. It is the fourth hurdle of health economics that presents the real challenge for many dentists (Fig 1-3).

In contrast, the private sector is able to address needs, aspirations and demands at an individual patient level which may be consistent with those at population level. The private sector service can be totally patient-focused because "the customer is king", although there may be a shared status where third party payers are involved.

The context of care delivery is further complicated by the fact that patients receive some types of care funded through the public sector and other services funded by private contract. The provider of these services now faces a further challenge – meeting and satisfying the varying regulatory requirements and satisfying the interpretation of quality imposed by all parties.

In the UK, this scenario is common where many practices provide services under the terms of the National Health Service (NHS) and private contract – so-called "mixing" of treatment.

A Changing Landscape

The approach to quality has changed over the years. Today's approach focuses on continuous quality improvement (CQI) and recognises evolving standards and the need for patient empowerment and involvement (Table 1-1).

Table 1-1 **Past and present approaches to quality**

Level of commitment	Yesterday's approach	Today's approach
Leadership commitment	Occasional review	Total quality management involving the entire practice
Emphasis of effort	Retrospective analysis	Proactive approach. Continuous quality improvement
Focus of effort	Retrospective inspection to catch error	Ongoing identification and improvement of faulty processes
Timing of effort	Retrospective analysis of quality indicators	Concurrent management of processes of care with built-in measures
Outcomes	Measure to acceptable standard	Measure against evolving standards

The aim of today's approach is to shift the mean standard of care over a period of time by a process of CQI (Fig 1-4 and Chapter 5).

Clinical Aspects

The meaning of quality is not only dependent on the observer's perspective, but also influenced by evolving standards, scientific advancements and changing societal values. Quality markers and indicators are time-sensitive. Today's guidance inspires and informs tomorrow's standards. Infection control standards in general dental practice are a prime example.

We are presented with research findings, clinical guidance and protocols and asked to adhere to certain standards. All the requirements have subtle differences in meaning and we should be aware of these if we are to implement them in a practical and relevant way.

Table 1-2 summarises the terminology used in clinical quality and gives a description of what it means.

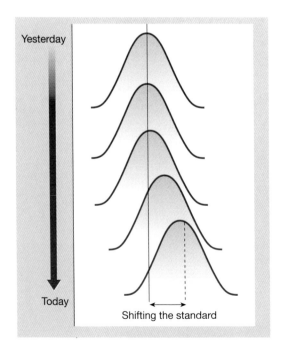

Shifting the standard

Fig 1-4 Shifting the mean standard of care.

Table 1-2 **Clinical quality vocabulary**

Clinical quality terms	Description
Standards	*Standards* are instruction documents that detail how a particular aspect of the project must be undertaken. The standard is absolute; there should be no variation.
Guidelines	Unlike Standards, *Guidelines* are not compulsory. They are intended to guide a project rather than dictate how it must be undertaken. Variations in your practice do not require formal approval.
Checklists	*Checklists* are useful as prompts and serve as a useful aide-memoire. They are particularly suitable for checking for compliance. A list of Health and Safety legislation is one example.
Templates	*Templates* are blank documents to be used in particular situations. They facilitate the recording of essential information that may be required for legislative or regulatory purposes. Templates for recording adverse incidents or complaints are two examples. Sample completed templates can serve as guides to what is required for satisfactory completion.
Procedures	*Procedures* outline the steps that should be undertaken in a particular activity. For example, a practice will have a procedure for welcoming a new patient to the practice.
Process	A *Process* is a description of how something works. It is often described graphically by means of a process map – commonly called a flow chart. A process also contains explanations of "why and how". In contrast a procedure is a list of steps – the "and when".
User guides	*User guides* provide the theory, principles and detailed instructions about how equipment should be used. They include technical information, definitions and the rationale for correct usage. Examples include user guides accompanying machines for dental radiography and film processing.
Methodology	A *Methodology* is a collection of processes, procedures, templates and other tools to guide the practice team through a particular activity. The clinical method for proving a full coverage metal-ceramic crown would involve the procedure of tooth preparation, the process of impression-taking and the fabrication of a provisional crown.

This is the *content* of everyday clinical care and it requires the *process* of care to deliver quality (Fig 1-5). This process is outlined in Fig 1-6.

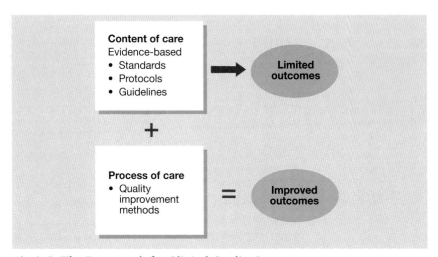

Fig 1-5 The Framework for Clinical Quality Improvement.
Adapted from: Batalden P, Stoltz P. A Framework for Continual Improvement in Healthcare. Joint Commission Journal on Quality Improvement. October 1997.

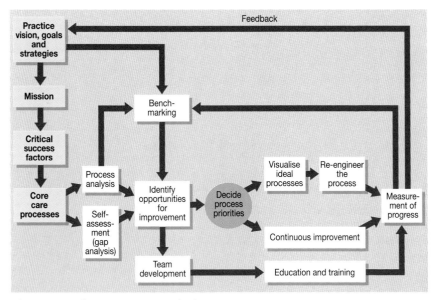

Fig 1-6 Quality in practice – the key processes.

Benefits

The benefits of implementing a quality programme are numerous. These are summarised in Fig 1-7.

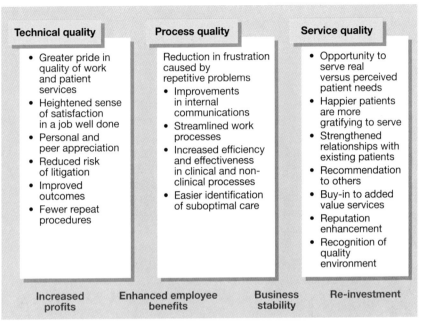

Technical quality

- Greater pride in quality of work and patient services
- Heightened sense of satisfaction in a job well done
- Personal and peer appreciation
- Reduced risk of litigation
- Improved outcomes
- Fewer repeat procedures

Process quality

Reduction in frustration caused by repetitive problems

- Improvements in internal communications
- Streamlined work processes
- Increased efficiency and effectiveness in clinical and non-clinical processes
- Easier identification of suboptimal care

Service quality

- Opportunity to serve real versus perceived patient needs
- Happier patients are more gratifying to serve
- Strengthened relationships with existing patients
- Recommendation to others
- Buy-in to added value services
- Reputation enhancement
- Recognition of quality environment

Increased profits   **Enhanced employee benefits**   **Business stability**   **Re-investment**

Fig 1-7 Benefits of quality initiatives in general dental practice.

References

Dutch National Council for Public Health. Nationale Raad voor de Volksgezondheid. Discussienota Begrippenkader Kwaliteit Beroepsuitoefening. Sept 1986;2.

Mindak MT. Service quality in dentistry: the role of the dental nurse. Br Dent J 1996;181:363-368.

Poorterman JHG. On quality of dental care: the development, validation and standardization of an index for the assessment of restorative care. PhD thesis, 1997.

Chapter 2
The Meaning of Quality

Aims

This chapter aims to explore the various definitions of quality and to define commonly used words and phrases. It also aims to summarise the valuable contributions made by some of the leading gurus of the quality movement.

Outcome

The reader should be familiar with a number of approaches to quality and the impact of some of the leading proponents in this field and how their views relate to general dental practice.

Introduction

Society has always been concerned about the quality of goods and services provided. Over the ages quality has developed as a discipline; the earliest paradigm of quality relying on the principle of *caveat emptor* (let the buyer beware) – an approach that placed the responsibility of appraising goods and services firmly with the user. The principles of quality control and total quality management came later with the industrial age, although there is evidence of conformance and control in ancient Rome. However, it was the post-industrial age that saw the development of the modern paradigm which impacts on the world as we see it today.

The American Society for Quality (ASQ) suggests that the term *"quality"* should not be used as a single term to express a degree of excellence in a comparative sense, nor should it be used in a quantitative sense for technical evaluations. These meanings, it suggests, should be communicated by a qualifying adjective.

A review of the literature suggests that there are numerous definitions of quality – almost as many as there are quality consultants. Hoyer and Hoyer (2001) surmised that these expert definitions of quality fall into two broad categories:

- Level one quality is a simple matter of producing products or delivering services, the measurable characteristics of which satisfy a fixed set of specifications that are usually numerically defined.
- Independent of any of their measurable characteristics, level two quality products and services are simply those that satisfy customer expectations for their use or consumption.

This approach is well suited to general dental practice where success is dependent on the delivery of quality care at both these levels.

The meaning and interpretation of quality is contextual; it depends on the nature of the service or product on offer and domain within which it is available. Some examples are listed in Table 2-1 and have certain themes in common, which are:

- Cost
- Time
- Customer experience
- Defect-free.

Table 2-1 **The contextualisation of quality**

Domain	The consumer view on quality indicators
Airlines	Safety, on-time, comfort, low-cost, good on-board food and drink
Healthcare	Correct diagnosis, minimum waiting time, safety, security, low cost
Restaurant food	Good food, fast delivery, comfortable environment, good atmosphere, polite service
Postal services	Fast delivery, reliable, low cost
Consumer products	Well made, fit for purpose, defect-free, good value
Mobile phone communication	Clear, fast, good coverage, low cost, design
Cars	Reliable, defect-free, faster, inclusion of extras, image and reputation of brand

Definitions

According to the American Institute of Medicine, quality is constituted by: "The degree to which health services for individuals and populations increase the likelihood of desired health outcomes and are consistent with current professional knowledge." It suggests that:

1. Quality performance and outcomes occur on a continuum, theoretically ranging from unacceptable to excellent.
2. The scope of inquiry is limited to the structure, process, and outcomes of care provided by the healthcare delivery system.
3. Quality may be assessed at multiple different levels.
4. The link between process and outcomes should be established.
5. Research evidence must be used to identify the services that improve health outcomes and in the absence of scientific evidence regarding effectiveness, professional consensus can be used to develop criteria.

In the UK, Donaldson and Muir Gray defined quality in healthcare as: "Doing the right thing, for the right person at the right time and getting it right first time." It is a definition that suits the practice of dentistry because it emphasises that there is more to quality than the quality of the technical outcome. For example, the quality of the outcome of root canal therapy on an upper molar may be undisputed, but if the root canal therapy has been the result of an incorrect or delayed diagnosis, then the patient has not received the "right thing at the right time". The root canal *therapy* may be excellent, but the quality of *care* may be less than satisfactory.

Another, more generally stated definition (European Committee for Standardization, 1994) holds that: "Quality is the totality of characteristics of an entity that bears on its ability to satisfy stated or implied needs." This allows both provider and patient expectations to be taken into account.

Øvretveit (1992) prefers a broader view, arguing that the scope of the above definition is limited by the fact that it considers the satisfaction of only those who receive the service and ignores those who do not. He defines quality as: "Fully meeting the needs of those who need the service most, at the lowest cost to the organisation, within limits and directives set by higher authorities and purchasers." Another interpretation introduces variance into the definition. Robert A. Broh observed that: "Quality is the degree of excellence at an acceptable price and the control of variability at an acceptable cost."

Table 2-2 **Some thoughts on the meaning of quality**

The meaning of quality

- Quality is the ongoing process of building and sustaining relationships by assessing, anticipating, and fulfilling stated and implied needs
- Quality is meeting the customer's needs in a way that exceeds the customer's expectations
- Quality is performance excellence as viewed by all stakeholders
- Quality is the customer's perception of the value of the supplier's work output
- Quality is the extent to which products, services, processes and relationships are free from defects, constraints and items that do not add value for customers
- Quality is when the customer returns and the product doesn't.

Karl Albrecht of Karl Albrecht International defines quality in two ways:

1. Objective quality is the degree of compliance of a process or its outcome with a predetermined set of criteria that are presumed essential to the ultimate value it provides. Example: the proper formulation of medicine.

2. Subjective quality is the level of perceived value reported by the person who benefits from a process or its outcome. It may subsume various intermediate quality measures, both objective and subjective. Example: the pain relief provided by medication.

During December 1999, readers of Quality Digest magazine were invited to submit their definitions of quality. Some of those definitions, which reflect the earlier discussions in this chapter, are shown in Table 2-2.

Terminology

Quality Assurance and Quality Improvement

The ASQ states the purpose of quality assurance is to: "Provide adequate confidence that a product or service will satisfy given needs." Quality assurance helps to identify outliers and usually involves external inspection and some form of accreditation.

Quality assurance is a widely used phrase and there are concerns about what it means. One is that the word *"assurance"* is a misnomer. Coster and Buetow make the point that whilst "quality can be protected and enhanced, it cannot be ensured". The other is that quality assurance sets minimum standards; this results in compliance to baseline thresholds, but does not instil the ethos of *continual* quality improvement.

A breach of those thresholds can lead to litigation, complaints and/or disciplinary action by the profession's regulatory bodies. It can also lead to a culture of "name, blame and shame" – a trend that healthcare organisations are keen to reverse. It is for these reasons that the preferred term amongst pundits is continuous quality improvement.

Continuous Quality Improvement (CQI)

Most problems are found in processes, and CQI aims to improve those processes through small, incremental changes (Fig 2-1). It has been defined as: "An approach to quality management that builds upon traditional quality assurance methods by emphasising the organisation and systems: focuses on 'process' rather than the individual; recognises both internal and external 'customers'; promotes the need for objective data to analyse and improve processes." (Source: Graham NO. Quality in Healthcare, 1995)

The key features of CQI are:
• Success is achieved through meeting the needs of patients.
• Most problems are found in processes, not in people.
• CQI does not seek to blame, but rather to improve processes.
• Unintended variation in processes can lead to unwanted variation in outcomes – this is addressed by reducing or eliminating such unwanted variations.

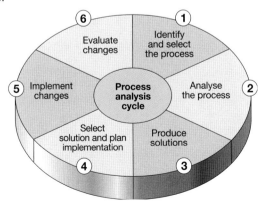

Fig 2-1 Analysing the process.

- It is possible to achieve continual improvement through small, incremental changes. CQI is itself evolutionary rather than revolutionary.
- CQI is most effective when it becomes a natural part of the way everyday work is done.
- It can be of limited value in situations where radical changes are required.

Attempts at CQI in practice can be frustrating. Some useful tips to bear in mind are:
- Define the problem before trying to solve it.
- Before you try to control a process, understand it.
- Before trying to control everything, first find out what is important and prioritise your efforts.
- Work on the processes that will have the biggest impact.
- Look at failure as a learning opportunity.

CQI is covered more fully in Chapter 5.

Quality assessment seeks to compare performance against explicit *a priori* criteria. It may be accomplished by observation, analysis, interview, a review of processes, evaluation of deliverables, measures, and identification of issues. It helps to highlight gaps in performance and identifies opportunities for improvement. It applies equally to clinical and non-clinical aspects of care within the practice and should lead to putting quality improvement initiatives in place.

Quality control is an operational technique that focuses on the process of producing the product or service with the intent of eliminating problems that might result in defects. Inspection is a quality control process. For example, careful checking of an impression before dispatch is an example of quality control. It does not prevent poor impressions being taken – the processes that lead to the final impression will do that.

Quality tools are instruments and/or techniques to support and improve the activities of process quality management and improvement. These are discussed more fully in Chapter 5.

Quality management is the sum of the management activities in the practice that determine the quality policy and bring about the quality improvement process.

Quality systems reflect the organisational structure, procedures, processes and resources needed to implement quality management.

Quality indicators are objective measures of the management process or outcomes of care and interventions in quantitative terms. The Royal College of General Practitioners in its publication, Quality Indicators in General Practice (2002), states that: "Quality indicators are at their most powerful when used as a mechanism for improving systems of care rather than judging performance."

They provide a measurable dimension of the quality of care. For example, a high percentage of patients returning for unscheduled appointments for pain and swelling after root canal therapy would be an indicator of the quality of endodontics therapy undertaken.

Quality Gurus

There is much that can be learned by studying the works of some the world's leading quality gurus and there is much that we can apply to everyday practice. Table 2-3 summarises those who have influenced the quality movement over the decades.

The same can be said of healthcare in general, a view that was endorsed in the September 2004 issue of Quality Progress, which carried the article "Can the Gurus' Concepts Cure Healthcare?" Written by four of America's leading experts, the article applied to modern healthcare the principles first advanced by Crosby, Deming, Feigenbaum and Juran.

These are legendary names in quality circles and a summary of their perspectives and implications for general practice are discussed here.

Table 2-3 **Leading quality figures**

1950s **The American influence**	Joseph M. Juran W. Edwards Deming Armand V. Feigenbaum
1950s and 1960s **The Japanese influence**	Dr Kaoru Ishikawa Shigeo Shingo
The western gurus of the 1970s and 1980s	Philip Crosby Tom Peters

Crosby

Philip Crosby is an American and a charismatic individual. An article in the Financial Times on 26 November 1986 described him thus: "Florida has provided him with a year-round tan. That, and his thinning hair and snappy dress gave him the look of a sunbelt Senator rather than a man from the quality department. He does have a campaign button in his lapel. It says ZD, of course, for Zero Defects."

And that is what he is best known for, namely the concepts of:
- Do it right first time
- Zero defects.

It is a level one definition.

Where he excelled was in finding a terminology for quality that was easily understood. His books, *Quality without Tears* and *Quality is Free*, are easy to read and he popularised the idea of the "cost of poor quality", emphasising how much it really costs to do things badly (see Chapter 9).

In his book, *Quality is Free,* Crosby notes the word quality is used to signify the relative worth of something in such phrases as "good quality" and "bad quality". He suggests that phrases such as "quality of life" have become meaningless clichés because: "Each listener assumes that the speaker means exactly what he or she, the listener, means by the phrase." It is for this reason that Crosby's view is that quality can be defined only by the phrase "conformance to requirements", which is a more objective interpretation.

To apply Crosby's philosophy, we must know what the requirements are in order to translate them into measurable characteristics. For example, we could define the characteristics of a quality crown on the basis of:
- marginal fit
- contact areas
- colour match
- occlusion
- emergence profile
- material characteristics.

Having established these requirements, we can then measure conformance. Crosby advocates that the system for creating quality is prevention of error and that the performance standard must be "zero defects" and not "that's close enough".

He lists the five characteristics of what he calls an "Eternally Successful Organisation" as:

1. People routinely do things right first time.
2. Change is anticipated and used to advantage.
3. Growth is consistent and profitable.
4. New products and services appear when needed.
5. Everyone is happy to work there.

It serves as a useful checklist for dental practices.

Peters

Tom Peters is best known for his writings on corporate management. In his third book, *Thriving on Chaos*, he describes some traits of the quality revolution he observed amongst top American companies. These are listed in Table 2-4.

Table 2-4 **The traits of quality** (continued over page)

Management obsession with quality	This stresses the importance of practical action to back up the emotional commitment, e.g. halving the number of re-work mechanics, never walking past shoddy goods
Measurement of quality	This should begin at the outset of the programme, should be displayed, and should be carried out by the participants
Quality is rewarded	Quality-based incentive compensation can cause an early breakthrough in top management's attitude
Everyone is trained for quality	Every person in the company should be extensively trained. Instruction in cause and effect analysis, statistical process control, and group interaction should be given to all
Multi-function teams	Quality Circles, or cross-functional teams such as Error Cause Removal or Corrective Action Teams should be introduced. Based on his experience, Peters favours cross-functional teams
Small is beautiful	According to Peters, there is no such thing as a small improvement. There is significance in the fact that a change has occurred

Table 2-4 **The traits of quality** (continued)

Create endless "Hawthorne" effects	This is the antidote to the 12–18 month doldrums. New goals, new themes, new events are the antidote. The Hawthorne effect refers to improvements in productivity or quality that result not because of changes to the working conditions, but because team members are being observed and this results in altered behaviours. So-called because of where the effects were first observed at the Hawthorne plants of Western Electric in Chicago
Parallel organisation structure devoted to quality improvement	This describes the creation of shadow quality teams and emphasises that it is a route through which hourly paid workers can progress
Everyone is involved	Suppliers especially, but distributors and customers too, must be part of the organisation's quality process. Joint improvement teams may be formed
When quality goes up, costs go down	Quality improvement is the primary source of cost reduction. The elementary force at work is simplification – of design, process or procedures for example
Quality improvement is a never-ending journey	All quality is relative. Each day, each product or service is getting relatively better or worse, but never stands still

Shigeo Shingo

Less well known in the West, Shingo's contribution to world prosperity was immense. His motto was that: "Those who are not satisfied will never make any progress." His paramount contribution was the development of poka-yoke ("mistake proofing") devices. He advocated stopping a process where a defect occurs in order to define the cause and prevent recurrence. Poka-yoke devices are discussed in *Risk Management in General Dental Practice*.

Ishikawa

Best known for his cause and effect diagram (see Chapter 3), this management leader made significant and specific advancements in quality improvement. It was Kaoru Ishikawa who also defined the concept of internal and external customers.

Table 2-5 **The Ishikawa way**

Quality begins with education and ends with education	A commitment to continuing professional development is paramount to creating a quality-driven dental practice
The first step in quality is to know the requirements of the patients	Understanding what is important to patients as consumers of dental services will help develop services in relation to patient expectations
The ideal state of quality control occurs when inspection of the work is no longer necessary	The culture and ethos within the practice is centred on quality. The team is empowered with this shared vision and quality checks are superfluous
Address the root cause of the problem, not the symptoms	The dentist who always runs late may blame the emergency patient but the root cause may be related to an ineffective appointment control system
Quality control is the responsibility of the entire team	The patient's perspective on quality is related to the clinical and non-clinical aspects of their care and experience. It is a team responsibility to ensure that the sum of individual experiences amounts to a total quality experience
Ninety-five per cent of problems in any practice can be solved with simple tools for analysis and problem solving	Practices should use tools such as significant event analysis and clinical audit to improve quality in the practice. These are discussed elsewhere in this text

We can learn from Ishikawa's philosophy and apply his thoughts to everyday practice as described in Table 2-5.

Feigenbaum

Dr Armand V. Feigenbaum's belief was that quality is a customer determination and as such is a level two definition. In his book, *Total Quality*

Control, he describes it as: "A customer's actual experience with the product or service measured against his or her requirements stated or unstated, conscious or merely sensed…" In other words, quality must be defined in terms of patient satisfaction. From his work, we must recognise that the needs and expectations of our patients change – so quality is dynamic. A feature of your practising style that wowed them yesterday may have become a baseline expectation today.

Applying Feigenbaum's principles, the two challenges in practice are to:
• determine what patients are willing to pay for the dentistry they need and/or want
• translate that information into the specification for our services.

The first is a management (marketing) function and the second a clinical function.

Feigenbaum's view is only partly applicable to dental practice because most patients cannot adequately judge the technical quality of clinical dentistry – a dental patient may be fully satisfied despite poor technical quality or vice versa. Given the patients' inability to judge clinical quality, they are more likely to rely on others to do it for them – this is where professional regulatory bodies have a role to play, as does accreditation and revalidation.

This begs the question, what are patients buying? The answer is they are often buying into a trust-based relationship. They may not know or understand the evidence-base for their prescribed treatment, but they rely on trust which leads them to believe that their dentist will apply his or her knowledge, understanding and skill for the good of the patient.

Until such time that patients are able to judge technical quality, they will judge quality primarily by what they can assess and experience – the environment and the service aspects of the care (see Chapter 9).

Deming
Dr W. Edwards Deming was one of the developers of the modern philosophy and methods associated with quality and quality improvement. Deming's philosophy is summarised in his famous "14 Points" listed opposite. These points have inspired significant changes among a number of leading US companies striving to compete in the world's increasingly competitive environment. Aspects of these 14 points are a useful source of discussion for general practitioners (Table 2-6).

Table 2-6 **Deming's 14 points** (continued over page)

Constancy of purpose	Deming advocated continual improvement of products and services with a long-term perspective in mind rather than focus on short-term profitability
The new philosophy	A new economic age demands a new management style. Deming said that defective workmanship was no longer acceptable if the West was to compete with the Japanese revolution in business
Cease dependence on mass inspection	Eliminate the need for inspection to achieve quality by building quality into the product in the first place
End lowest tender contracts	Deming advocated ending the practice of awarding business solely on the basis of the price tag – an interesting perspective for dentistry where public sector funded payment systems coexist with private arrangements. He suggested reducing the number of suppliers for the same item to establish loyalty and trust
Improve every process	Improve constantly and forever every process for planning, production and service. Search continually for problems in order to improve every activity in the company and to improve quality
Institute on-the-job training	Deming advocated on-the-job training methods for all to ensure that people kept pace with changes in materials, technology and techniques
Institute leadership	Let the leaders take responsibility for quality
Drive out fear	This can be achieved by encouraging two-way conversation and creating a no blame environment. It is interesting to note that this is something which healthcare providers are implementing through clinical governance
Break down barriers	Deming encouraged teamwork to avoid barriers between different units within an organisation

Table 2-6 **Deming's 14 points** (continued)

Eliminate exhortations	Eliminate the use of slogans, posters and exhortations for the workforce, demanding Zero Defects and new levels of productivity, without providing methods. Such exhortations only create adversarial relationships; the bulk of the causes of low quality and low productivity belong to the system, and thus lie beyond the power of the workforce
Eliminate arbitrary numerical targets	Eliminate work standards that prescribe quotas for the workforce
Permit pride of workmanship	Remove the barriers that rob hourly workers, and people in management, of their right to pride of workmanship. This implies, among other things, abolition of the annual merit rating (appraisal of performance) and of Management by Objective. Again, the responsibility of commissioning managers must be changed from sheer numbers to quality
Encourage education	A vigorous programme of education should be encouraged – Deming believed that competitive advantage had its roots in knowledge
Top management commitment and action	Clearly define top management's permanent commitment to ever-improving quality and productivity, and their obligation to implement all of these principles

Juran

Joseph M. Juran is considered by many to be the greatest quality thinker of the last century. His books and publications have been translated into a dozen languages and he has received countless accolades, honours and medals. *Juran's Quality Handbook* – now in its fifth edition – remains an international favourite.

He states that there are no short cuts to quality. Juran's view on quality integrates level one and level two approaches. His definition of quality is "fitness for use". In other words, quality is taken to be present when the products or services fulfil the purpose for which they were produced (Fig 2-2).

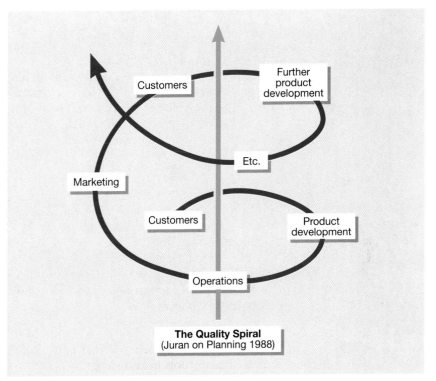

Fig 2-2 Juran's quality spiral.

This definition is not without its problems because expectations may vary with the provider and different types of customers. So whether a product performs the functions for which it was designed may ultimately depend on the expectations of functions of a particular product. But this definition of quality moves the focus closer to the user or customer.

This definition requires that the needs of the customer are well understood and that the products are carefully tested to perform as expected.

Juran's prescription for quality focuses on three processes (Fig 2-3). His quality trilogy focuses on:
• Quality planning – this is about building quality into a process from the outset.
• Quality control – this is concerned with maintaining the performance of a process.

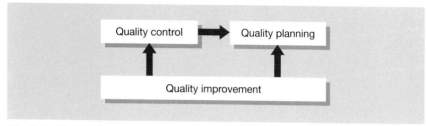

Fig 2-3 The quality trilogy.

- Quality improvement – this is about changing a process to achieve unprecedented levels of performance.

Advising the CEO of Massachusetts Respiratory Hospital on quality, Juran's advice was to "staple yourself to the process", by which he meant study, analyse and dissect the process every step of the way.

Summary

The synthesis of data from quality experts leads us to the nine dimensions of quality, which have been identified as:

1. Technical performance: The degree to which the tasks carried out by health workers and facilities meet expectations of technical quality (i.e. adherence to standards).
2. Access to services: The degree to which healthcare services are unrestricted by geographic, economic, social, organisational, or linguistic barriers.
3. Effectiveness of care: The degree to which desired results (outcomes) of care are achieved.
4. Efficiency of service delivery: The ratio of the outputs of services to the associated costs of producing those services.
5. Interpersonal relations: Trust, respect, confidentiality, courtesy, responsiveness, empathy, effective listening, and communication between providers and clients.
6. Continuity of services: Delivery of care by the same healthcare provider throughout the course of care (when appropriate) and appropriate and timely referral and communication between providers.
7. Safety: The degree to which the risks of injury, infection, or other harmful side effects are minimised.
8. Physical infrastructure and comfort: The physical appearance of the facility, cleanliness, comfort, privacy, and other aspects that are important to clients.

9. Choice: As appropriate and feasible, client choice of provider, insurance plan, or treatment.

Quality means different things to different people. In can be defined according to these different perspectives (Table 2-7).

Table 2-7 **Dimensions of quality** (after Garvin)

1. Patient-based	Fitness for intended use, meeting customer expectations
2. Technical basis	Conforming to design, specifications or requirements, having no defects
3. Product-based	The product has something that adds value that other similar products do not
4. Value-based	The product is the best combination of price and features. A quality product is one that provides performance at an acceptable price or conformance at an acceptable cost
5. Transcendent	It is not clear what it is, but it is something good

References

Albrecht K. The only thing that matters. New York: HarperCollins, 1992.

American Society for Quality, www.asq.org

Broh RA. Managing quality for higher profits: a guide for business executives and quality managers. New York: McGraw-Hill, 1982.

Coster G, Buetow S. Quality in the New Zealand Health System. Background Paper to the National Health Committee. National Health Committee, Sept 2001.

Crosby P. Quality is Free: the art of making quality certain. Signet Books, 1993.

Crosby P. Quality without tears. New York: McGraw-Hill, 1995.

Donaldson LJ, Muir Gray JA. Clinical governance: a quality duty for health organisations. Qual Health Care 1998;7:suppl.S37-S44.

European Committee for Standardization (www.cenorm.be), 1994.

Feigenbaum AV. Total Quality Control. 4th edn. New York: McGraw-Hill, 2004.

Garvin DA. Managing Quality: the strategic and competitive edge. New York: Free Press, 1988.

Graham NO. Quality in Healthcare. Theory, application and evolution. Gaithersburg MD: Aspen Publication, 1995.

Hoyer RW, Hoyer BBY. What Is Quality? Qual Progress J 2001;34(7):52-62.

Juran JM. Juran's Quality Handbook. 5th edn. New York: McGraw-Hill, 1998.

Nielsen DM, Merry MD, Schyve PM, Bisognano M. Can the Gurus' Concepts Cure Healthcare? Qual Progress J 2004;37(9):25-34.

Øvretveit J. Health Service Quality: An introduction to quality methods for health services. Oxford: Blackwell Science, 1992.

Peters T. Thriving on Chaos. New York: HarperCollins, 1991.

Quality Digest Magazine, Paton Press, December 1999.

The Royal College of General Practitioners. Quality Indicators in General Practice. Policy Statement, 2002.

Chapter 3

Quality Concepts

Aim

The aim of this chapter is to review some of the common quality concepts and frameworks and how they can be used to help develop quality initiatives in everyday practice.

Outcome

The reader should be familiar with some key quality concepts that can have an impact on the implementation of a quality programme in general dental practice.

Introduction

Of the many quality assessment frameworks that exist, Donabedian's (1966) concept is perhaps the most applicable to all aspects of general dental practice. In his classic text on healthcare quality, Avedis Donabedian presents a fundamental concept regarding the nature of any activity designed to produce a consistent result. The concept (Fig 3-1) has three attributes:
1. Structure
2. Process
3. Outcome.

Structure

This relates to the practice facilities, equipment, the team members, and organisation available for the provision of care.

Process

This pertains to the procedures and protocols that the dental team have to conform to so as to ensure appropriate and adequate delivery of dental services. Every activity in the dental practice is part of a process and the process itself includes an input, an action and an output – the process for instrument decontamination and sterilisation provides a good example.

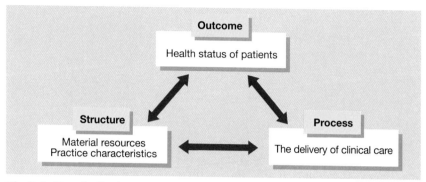

Fig 3-1 Donabedian's concept.

Most processes are not perfect. There is generally some wasted effort, or lost time, or wastage, or miscommunication, or redoing. These problems all have costs – some small, and some great. By focusing on processes, rather than on the individuals involved in the process, we get much more rapid, substantial improvements. A good example is preparing dental materials – the properties of many dental materials are affected by measuring and mixing techniques but important aspects of the process may be omitted – usually because manufacturer's instructions have not been followed.

Outcome

This denotes the effects of care on a patient's dental health status. Both positive and negative outcomes should be studied to analyse the processes that led to them. Donabedian noted that: "Although outcomes might indicate good or bad care in the aggregate, they do not give an insight into the nature and location of the deficiencies or strengths to which the outcome might be attributed."

The *quality* of an output is an evaluation. It is an individual's personal judgement of some set of attributes of the output. It results from the individual's perceptions of the output and is rooted within the individual's personal frame of reference. It is often a *relative* term with no fixed unit of measurement.

This means that it is a unit-less value system and therefore can only be assessed by comparison to other similar items. The corollary to this argument is that the terms "good" and "bad" quality have no real meaning, but the terms "better" or "worse" quality do because of the comparative nature of the perception. The comparisons we make in clinical practice will be based on our past personal experiences and prejudices – those prejudices in turn and in part at least being determined by a host of external influences. From the patient's point of view, the personal element will be expressed as an "expectation"; when positive expectations are met, quality is judged to be acceptable, and when expectations are exceeded, then quality is judged to be excellent. This is explored further in Chapter 7.

Looking at outcomes in isolation, without examining the processes that lead to them, is of limited value, but nonetheless this is what often happens in a practice. A crown does not fit and "someone" is to blame or a remake is indicated without an analysis of the "why"? The "5-why technique" of root cause analysis discussed in *Risk Management in General Dental Practice* is recommended here.

Outcomes should be analysed in relation to their causal antecedents. Clinical outcomes are generally regarded as falling into one or more of the following categories:

- Functional status and wellbeing
- Conventional physiological and biomedical measurements
- Costs of healthcare delivery
- Patient satisfaction with care.

The cost of unacceptable outcomes is covered in Chapter 10.

Linking Structure and Process

Structure has an impact on *outcome* mainly through the *process* of care. Each of these three dimensions can be assessed separately or in combination. The question arises whether, if structure and process are suitably addressed, the patient can be assured of a satisfactory outcome? In theory, the answer is yes. The clinical example in Fig 3-2 demonstrates the principle. If all the stages of the process are followed and the required materials are available to support these processes, the outcome is highly satisfactory. The final product is defect-free and, providing it meets or, preferably, exceeds the patient's expectations will be perceived as a quality outcome by all the stakeholders (including the dental technician).

In reality, we know that outcomes can be affected by patient behaviour, for which the clinician cannot always be held responsible. The progression of periodontal disease in a non- or partially-compliant patient is a good example.

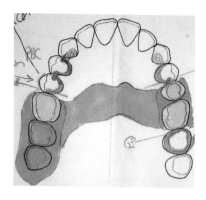

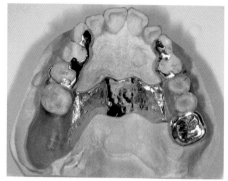

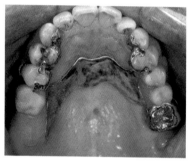

Fig 3-2 From design to fit: a synergy of structure and process.

It is also true that a poor outcome does not always result every time there is an error in the provision of care. We can all cite cases of root canal therapy, which radiographically appears inadequate (for whatever reason), but which has been *in situ* for many years and does not appear to have compromised the long-term prognosis of the treated tooth. For this reason, it is argued that an assessment of quality should depend more on process data than on outcome data (Fig 3-3).

A patient who attends for a tooth extraction may be the subject of a poor process which results in the successful outcome, namely the tooth has been extracted. If the process of extraction lasted 30 minutes because of misapplication of instrument/technique, an outcome measure will not identify it. If a different process had been applied, then the same outcome could have been achieved in say 10 minutes – a process measure would therefore be far more valuable in this situation. In other words, "getting there in the end" is not what quality is about.

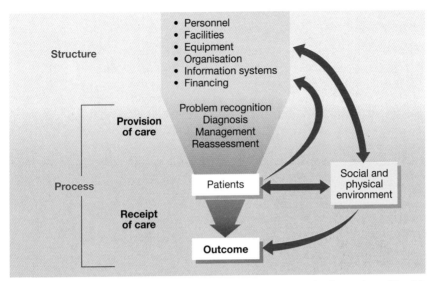

Fig 3-3 Relations of structure and process components in dynamics of health outcome. Modified from Starfield (1974).

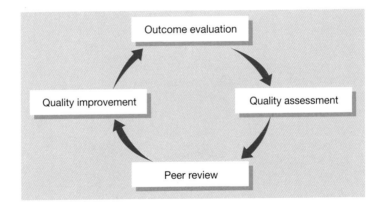

Fig 3-4
Outcome
assess-
ment.

Peer Review

Aspects of the structure, process and outcomes in clinical practice are best examined amongst professional colleagues by the process of peer review. It ensures that the loop between quality assessment and quality improvement is closed and will result in improved standards of care for patients by encouraging changes in clinical practice (Fig 3-4).

Benchmarking

The word "benchmark" was first used by the Xerox Corporation in the 1970s. The word entered the quality lexicon in 1990 when Xerox won the acclaimed Malcolm Baldridge National Quality Award in 1990. It was described as: "The continuous process of measuring products, services, and practices against the company's toughest competitors or those companies renowned as industry leaders." We can define it as the process of identifying, understanding and adapting outstanding practices from a variety of sources to help your practice to improve its performance. It means using someone else's successful process as a measure of desired achievement for a defined activity. It looks outward to find best practice and then measures your practice's operations and processes against those standards.

In our everyday world, benchmarks are something to measure up to. We benchmark our children's growth against norms for age groups, our salaries against our peers, our intelligence against established norms, our sporting aspirations against standards of fellow enthusiasts, and our professional services against those of our competitors.

Almost all practice processes can be benchmarked – the benchmark is the measure by which that system or process is judged to be successful or effective.

The four common types of benchmarking are:
- Internal
- Competitive
- External
- Generic process.

The difference reflects the information source of the innovation.

If a practising dentist wishes to review a particular aspect of his clinical practice, he is able to do this by talking to and/or observing other dentists in the same practice to identify *internal* innovations, or may seek views from other practices to discover *external* sources of innovation.

A variation on external benchmarking is international benchmarking where partners are sought from other countries – a trend that is observable in the UK where some US cosmetically centred practices are benchmark partners to some in the UK. It should be noted that not all processes are transferable from one environment to another.

Table 3-1 **Benchmarking in practice**

Benchmarking	How it should be used
Useful for applying good ideas from others	1. Identify best practice guidance from other practices and professional organisations
Helps to develop your plans for quality improvement within your practice	2. Select the superior performers
	3. Collect and analyse data
Increases understanding of what is known to work after testing	4. Improve
	5. Take corrective action if performance does not meet goals

If you want to consider the way new patients are greeted and handled, then you may decide to review the practices of say a hotel group known for its excellent customer service – this would reflect a *generic* approach.

In *competitive* benchmarking, the partners are drawn from the same sector. For example, some accountants that specialise in working with dentists offer their clients benchmark ratios for business expenditure and cost control purposes. A practice management consultant may do the same with service-orientated benchmarks. It is common for this type of benchmarking to be undertaken by third parties to protect confidentiality.

In summary, benchmarking is a technique for learning from others' successes in an area where the team is trying to make improvements (Table 3-1). An example of the benchmark standard developed for the National Health Service (NHS) is shown in Fig 3-5.

The toolkit includes:
• an overall patient-focused outcome that expresses what patients and/or carers want from care in a particular area of practice
• a number of factors that need to be considered in order to achieve the overall patient-focused outcome.

Each factor consists of:
• a patient-focused benchmark of best practice which is placed at the extreme right of the continuum
• a continuum between poor and best practice.

Agreed patient-focused outcome

Patients and carers experience effective communication, sensitive to their individual needs and preferences, that promotes high-quality care for the patient

	Factor	Benchmark of best practice
1.	Interpersonal skills	All healthcare personnel demonstrate effective interpersonal skills when communicating with patients and/or carers
2.	Opportunity for communication	Communication takes place at a time and in an environment that is acceptable to all parties
3.	Assessment of communication needs	All patients' and/or carers' communication needs are assessed on initial contact and are regularly reassessed. Additional communication support is negotiated and provided when a need is identified
4.	Information sharing	Information that is accessible, acceptable, up to date and meets the needs of individuals is shared actively and consistently with all patients and/or carers and widely promoted across all communities
5.	Resources to aid communication and understanding	Appropriate and effective methods of communication are used actively to promote understanding between patients and/or carers and healthcare personnel
6.	Assessment to identity principal carer	The principal carer is identified at all times and an assessment is made with them of their needs, involvement, willingness and ability to collaborate with practitioners in order to provide care
7.	Empowerment to perform role	All patients and/or carers are continuously supported and fully enabled to perform their role safely
8.	Coordination of care	All care providers communicate fully and effectively with each other to ensure that patients and/or carers benefit from a comprehensive plan of care which is regularly updated and evaluated
9.	Empowerment to communicate needs	All patients and/or carers are enabled to communicate their individual needs and preferences at all times
10.	Valuing the patients' and/or carers' expertise and contribution	Effective communication ensures and demonstrates that the patients' and/or carers' expert contribution to patient care is valued, recorded and informs both patient care and healthcare personnel education with ongoing review
11.	Training needs	All the patients' and/or carers' information, support and training needs are jointly identified, agreed, met and regularly reviewed

Fig 3-5 Patient-focused outcomes and best practice benchmarks.

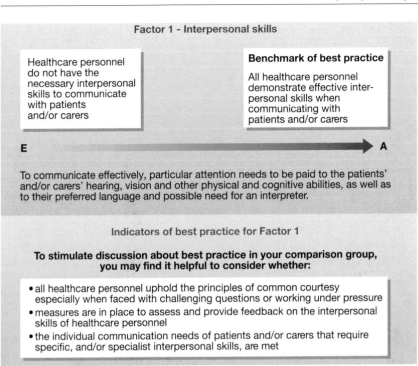

Fig 3-6 Using indicators of best practice for the first factor listed in Fig 3-5. Source: Benchmark of Best Practice: Effective Communication in Essence of Care. In: Patient Focused Benchmarks for Clinical Governance. Modernisation Agency. Dept. of Health April 2003.

The benchmark for each factor guides users towards best practice indicators for best practice identified by patients, carers and professionals that support the attainment of best practice. A self-assessment rating is then applied on a visual analogue scale from A-E, after discussion about the indicators (Fig 3-6).

Kaizen

In many ways, the Kaizen concept is a philosophy. Originally a Buddhist term and widely recognised in Japanese corporations for almost 50 years, Kaizen means "renew the heart and make it good". It demands a change in "the heart of the dental practice" – in other words it is culture, structure and vision.

Kaizen is about ongoing, continuous improvement. It focuses on small incremental changes on a continuous basis as opposed to radical change or a revolution – in other words, you should not look for radical changes but rely on a day-by-day common sense approach to improving and being better.

Masaaki Imai is the chairman and founder of the Kaizen Institute. It was Imai who came up with the line: "If you don't have the money, use your brains, if you don't have the brains ... sweat it out." His 1986 book, *Kaizen – The Key to Japan's Competitive Success*, has been translated into 14 languages. In it, he describes Kaizen as meaning: "Continuing improvement in personal life, home life, social life, and working life." When applied to the workplace Kaizen means continuing improvement involving everyone – clinicians and administrators alike.

Table 3-2 **The principles of Kaizen** (continued over page)

1. Discard conventional fixed ideas	Conventional, fixed ideas would suggest that it is not necessary to continue learning throughout our lives. The entire ethos of continuing professional development is to advance the frontiers of knowledge.
2. Think of how to do it, not why it cannot be done	The pessimist will create all kinds of reasons that something can't be done. The optimistic, forward thinker, on the other hand, knows that "if the why is strong enough, the how will come." Focus on the outcome and how it can be accomplished.
3. Do not make excuses	Start by questioning current practices. Making excuses for not doing something is easy. Again, focus on the outcome. Then, take action. There is no excuse for not trying something.
4. Do not seek perfection	If we all waited for perfection, we'd still be reading by candlelight and riding horses to work. Once you get to a certain point (whether it is 50% or 80%, or another number that makes sense), then run with it. In other words, take action. Then, adjust as you go along. This is a management doctrine, not a clinical guideline!

Table 3-2 **The principles of Kaizen** (continued)

5. Correct it right away, if you make a mistake	Acknowledge that the mistake happened, especially when it affects other people, and then correct it with point 4 above in mind. This is consistent with reflective practice.
6. Do not just spend money for Kaizen, use your wisdom	It is not enough to simply to read a book, watch a DVD, or attend a seminar. These may be essential first steps, but *action* is key. Learn and take action based on what you have learned. In other words, walk the talk.
7. Wisdom is brought out when faced with hardship	Challenges are usually undesirable, but they can be tremendous learning opportunities. Obstacles will present themselves, and you will be a better person for having done what it took to overcome them.
8. Ask "why" five times and seek root causes	The question "why" is extremely powerful. The question "why" can serve to either strengthen our conviction about something, and/or to discover that it really was not as important as we thought it was. At a minimum, it helps us to get to the root of the issue.
9. Seek the wisdom of ten people rather than the knowledge of one	Much has been written about the power of group thinking. Whether it involves seeking one or two other people's opinions or holding a meeting with colleagues, there is power in numbers. If you want to find out how to be successful at something, ask someone who has already done it. Better still, gather several people who have already done it.
10. Kaizen ideas are infinite	There is no limit to what is achievable with the Kaizen mindset of quality improvement. "Kaizen", said Imai in an interview with a journalist, "should be in your thought, word and deed."

The word *gemba* (literal meaning "real place"), often appears alongside the Kaizen concept and Imai has broadened its meaning to include any on-the-spot location where real actions and transactions take place. In his 1997 book, *Gemba Kaizen – A commonsense low cost approach to management,* he advocates the use of every on-the-spot opportunity for improvement. Imai's Kaizen principles are summarised in Table 3-2.

ISO 9000

The International Organization for Standardization is the world's largest developer of standards. ISO 9000 has become an international reference for quality requirements in business-to-business dealings. The ISO 9000 family of international quality management standards and guidelines has earned a global reputation as the basis for establishing quality management systems.

The increasing popularity of ISO 9000 certification has brought to the fore another significant definition of quality. ISO 9000-certified businesses are measured against public notions of quality rather than the one adopted by ISO itself. ISO 9000 defines quality as: "A totality of characteristics of an entity that bears on its ability to meet the stated and unstated needs" (ISO 8402: 1994). This definition is quite unlike the others. It refers to the characteristics of an organisation – to quality organisations, not products.

The existence of policies, procedures, instructions, records and constant reviews ensures that products conform to specifications. While the ultimate objective is customer satisfaction, the focus is on the organisational characteristics – the vehicle for producing quality products.

The quality principles advocated by ISO and how they relate to general dental practice are summarised in Table 3-3.

The reader is referred to www.iso.org for more details about ISO certification.

Investors in People

It is generally regarded that people are any organisation's greatest asset. To succeed in the business of dentistry, the team has to perform well, which requires the right knowledge, skills and attitude to work effectively and efficiently.

Table 3-3 **ISO principles and their application in general dental practice**

Customer focus	• Patient-focused care • The patient experience • Clinical risk reduction programmes
Leadership	• Formulation of practice policy • Leadership skill development
Involvement of people	• Learning from complaints • Patient satisfaction surveys
Process approach	• Quality improvement processes • Peer review • Clinical audit • Risk management
System approach to management	• Put in place management systems to allow practice to function • Systems to investigate significant events • Integration of processes into systems
Continual improvement	• Implementation of professional development programmes • Dealing with poor performance • Personal learning plans for team members
Factual approach to decision making	• Evidence-based practice • Use of high-quality data to monitor clinical care • Dissemination of good ideas
Mutually beneficial customer-supplier relationships	• Maintenance of internal and external relationships • Effective use of resources

The Investors in People (IIP) Standard is a quality framework that can help in this quest. The IIP approach is based on the PDCA cycle, which is discussed in Chapter 5. The process is summarised in Fig 3-7. The IIP standards framework comprises three fundamental principles with the 10 indicators shown in Fig 3-7.

41

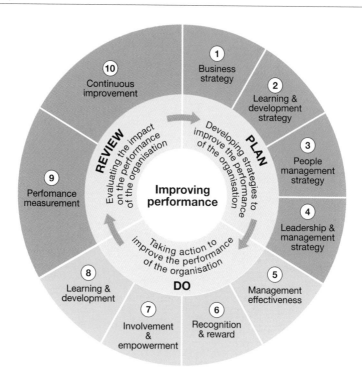

Fig 3-7 The Investors in People approach.

The evidence required to support the indicators is listed in Fig 3-8 (Source: Investors in People). The achievement of the standard is an example of external validation (see Table 4-5 in Chapter 4). Successful practices are awarded a plaque to indicate their achievement, Fig 3-9 (page 45).

The People vs. Systems Concept

The people vs. systems debate continues amongst quality consultants. One of the driving elements of Mankind seems to be the desire to improve – and without this, it could be argued that the threat of extinction intensifies. The same is true of clinical practice – the pursuit of continuous quality improvement must deliver an inner satisfaction in the work we do. Without this we are condemned to perpetual dissatisfaction.

Prin-ciples	Indicators	Evidence requirements
An Investor in People develops effective strategies to improve the performance of the organisation through its people. **Developing strategies to improve the performance of the organisation**	**1** A strategy for improving the performance of the organisation is clearly defined and understood.	1 Top managers make sure the organisation has a clear purpose and vision supported by a strategy for improving its performance. 2 Top managers make sure the organisation has a business plan with measurable performance objectives. 3 Top managers make sure there are constructive relationships with representative groups (where they exist) and the groups are consulted when developing the organisation's business plan. 4 Managers can describe how they involve people when developing the organisation's business plan and when agreeing team and individual objectives. 5 People who are members of representative groups can confirm that top managers make sure there are constructive relationships with the groups and they are consulted when developing the organisation's business plan. 6 People can explain the objectives of their team and the organisation at a level that is appropriate to their role, and can describe how they are expected to contribute to developing and achieving them.
	2 Learning and development is planned to achieve the organisation's objectives.	1 Top managers can explain the organisation's learning and development needs, the plans and resources in place to meet them, how these link to achieving specific objectives and how the impact will be evaluated. 2 Managers can explain team learning and development needs, the activities planned to meet them, how these link to achieving specific team objectives and how the impact will be evaluated. 3 People can describe how they are involved in identifying their learning and development needs and the activities planned to meet them. 4 People can explain what their learning and development activities should achieve for them, their team and the organisation.
	3 Strategies for managing people are designed to promote equality of opportunity in the development of the organisation's people.	1 Top managers can describe strategies they have in place to create an environment where everyone is encouraged to contribute ideas to improve their own and other people's performance. 2 Top managers recognise the different needs of people and can describe strategies they have in place to make sure everyone has appropriate and fair access to the support they need and there is equality of opportunity for people to learn and develop which will improve their performance. 3 Managers recognise the different needs of people and can describe how they make sure everyone has appropriate and fair access to the support they need and there is equality of opportunity for people to learn and develop which will improve their performance. 4 People believe managers are genuinely committed to making sure everyone has appropriate and fair access to the support they need and there is equality of opportunity for them to learn and develop which will improve their performance. 5 People can give examples of how they have been encouraged to contribute ideas to improve their own and other people's performance.
	4 The capabilities managers need to lead, manage and develop people effectively are clearly defined and understood.	1 Top managers can describe the knowledge, skills and behaviours managers need to lead, manage and develop people effectively, and the plans they have in place to make sure managers have these capabilities. 2 Managers can describe the knowledge, skills and behaviours they need to lead, manage and develop people effectively. 3 People can describe what their manager should be doing to lead, manage and develop them effectively.

Fig 3-8 The principles, indicators and evidence requirements of IIP (cont. over page).

Principles	Indicators	Evidence requirements
Taking action to improve the performance of the organisation — An Investor in People takes effective action to improve the performance of the organisation through its people.	**(5)** Managers are effective in leading, managing and developing people.	1 Managers can explain how they are effective in leading, managing and developing people. 2 Managers can give examples of how they give people constructive feedback on their performance regularly and when appropriate. 3 People can explain how their managers are effective in leading, managing and developing them. 4 People can give examples of how they receive constructive feedback on their performance regularly and when appropriate.
	(6) People's contribution to the organisation is recognised and valued.	1 Managers can give examples of how they recognise and value people's individual contribution to the organisation. 2 People can describe how they contribute to the organisation and believe they make a positive difference to its performance. 3 People can describe how their contribution to the organisation is recognised and valued.
	(7) People are encouraged to take ownership and responsibility by being involved in decision-making.	1 Managers can describe how they promote a sense of ownership and responsibility by encouraging people to be involved in decision-making, both individually and through representative groups, where they exist. 2 People can describe how they are encouraged to be involved in decision-making that affects the performance of individuals, teams and the organisation, at a level that is appropriate to their role. 3 People can describe how they are encouraged to take ownership and responsibility for decisions that affect the performance of individuals, teams and the organisation, at a level that is appropriate to their role.
	(8) People learn and develop effectively.	1 Managers can describe how they make sure people's learning and development needs are met. 2 People can describe how their learning and development needs have been met, what they have learnt and how they have applied this in their role. 3 People who are new to the organisation, and those new to a role, can describe how their induction has helped them to perform effectively.
Evaluating the impact on the performance of the organisation — An Investor in People can demonstrate the impact of its investment in people on the performance of the organisation	**(9)** Investment in people improves the performance of the organisation.	1 Top managers can describe the organisation's overall investment of time, money and resources in learning and development. 2 Top managers can explain, and quantify where appropriate, how learning and development has improved the performance of the organisation. 3 Top managers can describe how the evaluation of their investment in people is used to develop their strategy for improving the performance of the organisation. 4 Managers can give examples of how learning and development has improved the performance of their team and the organisation. 5 People can give examples of how learning and development has improved their performance, the performance of their team and that of the organisation.
	(10) Improvements are continually made to the way people are managed and developed.	1 Top managers can give examples of how the evaluation of their investment in people has resulted in improvements in the organisation's strategy for managing and developing people. 2 Managers can give examples of improvements they have made to the way they manage and develop people. 3 People can give examples of improvements that have been made to the way the organisation manages and develops its people.

Fig 3-8 The principles, indicators and evidence requirements of IIP (continued).

Systemic ineffectiveness arises when members of the team work well *alone,* but not as part of a *team.* Personal ineffectiveness arises when people are not performing to their potential. Many dentists will know from their experience of running practices that personal ineffectiveness creates a drag on practice systems, and bad systems clearly engender less effective people – this is the vicious circle of declining effectiveness. In contrast, virtuous circles also exist, in which people and systems continually improve – business and clinical performance can be turned around under new management and leadership.

In Chapter 2, we discussed the contribution of Deming and Juran and their belief that the overwhelming majority of quality failures is the result of systemic problems, not individual shortcomings. Recently, this view has been endorsed in many areas of healthcare with particular reference to both error and risk management. The author has elected not to reconsider this aspect of quality as it has been covered in a previous title in this series, *Risk Management in General Dental Practice.*

People and systems must work in tandem to achieve optimum results. It was Gandhi who warned that to wish for a system so perfect was flawed because no one will need to be good.

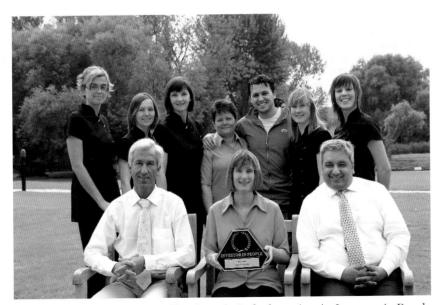

Fig 3-9 The practice team at Iffley Dental, Oxford, receives its Investors in People Award (2006).

References

Donabedian A. Evaluating the quality of medical care. Milbank Memorial Fund Quarterly: Health and Society 1966;44:166-203.

Imai M. Gemba Kaizen: a commonsense low cost approach to management. New York: McGraw-Hill, 1997.

Imai M. Kaizen: the Key to Japan's Competitive Success. Am Soc Qual, 1986.

Starfield B. Measurement of Outcome: A proposed scheme. The Milbank Memorial Fund Quarterly: Health and Society 1974;52:39-50.

Chapter 4
The Challenge of Measurement

Aims

This chapter aims to summarise the different ways in which quality can be measured and to identify the tools and techniques available to measure quality in practice. It also aims to highlight some of the challenges of measurement.

Outcome

After reading this chapter, the reader should better understand the dilemmas associated with measuring quality and be familiar with a number of tools that can help with quality measurement.

Introduction

What gets measured gets done. It is a dictum from the earliest of civilisations and has been at the heart of all human endeavour and discovery; Egyptian wall paintings from around 1450 BC show evidence of measurement and inspection.

In practice, measurement tools enable us to measure many variables, from defects in our clinical procedures (impressions and casts for example), to costs in relation to revenue. Key performance measures need to be easily understood, cost effective to measure, should not distort what is being measured and be aligned with the objectives of the management and processes that they are measuring. We need to measure so that we know that changes made in clinical practice actually lead to improvements. A feature of a measure is that it is precise, objective and consistent so that two individuals should obtain the same value as a result of carrying out the same measurement.

Quality should be measured based upon the exchange that is occurring. Depending on the objectives, it may be measured differently for the exchange between the commissioner and its provider, the provider and the patient and the provider and his/her peers. This is highly relevant where there is a shift away from nationally managed services to locally managed services.

Terminology

A *measure* is an operation for deriving a numerical representation: "If we put someone on a scale, we can *measure* how many kilos they weigh."

A *measurement* is the discrete implementation of the measure: "If we put me on a scale, we can see that I am about 90 kilos."

A *metric* is an interpretation of a measure; it assigns meaning to the number provided by a measure. It is reflected in the statement: "I *weigh* 90 kilos."

Performance measures should be developed so that they are reliable and valid.

Reliability

A reliable measure will give the same result every time that it is applied to the same aspect of healthcare. A thermometer is a reliable measure – it will show the same temperature each time it is used to measure the temperature in a particular location in a living room (provided the temperature has not changed). The latest generation of apex locators is reliable for the determination of working length during endodontic procedures – they will give the same reading if the reading is repeated. In contrast, electric pulp testers, for example, may not be quite as reliable.

Validity

A valid measure will be reliable and will also measure the intended aspect. In the case of the thermometer, the position of the thermometer should measure ambient temperature in the room, but if placed by an open window, will not provide a valid measurement.

Example

A practice may record the number of written complaints it has received – for example, seven over the course of a year. The measure is reliable (no matter how many times you count the letters, there will be seven), but it is not valid because it does not relate the number of complaints received to the total number of patients seen, and/or the number of completed courses of treatment. A ratio is required for the measure to be valid. If the definition of a "complaint" is unclear, then the reliability of the measure is also compromised. This is particularly important for inter-practice comparisons, because some queries may be perceived as complaints and vice versa.

Quality Indicators

The pursuit of quality in everyday practice is a long and never-ending journey; quality indicators are the signposts along that journey. In Chapter 1, quality indicators were defined as units of information which reflect, directly or indirectly, the performance of the practice in maintaining or increasing the wellbeing of its patients. By definition, indicators are imprecise. They are tools that are useful to clinicians and managers but, like any tool, the benefits from their use come from the way they are applied and also the purpose for which they are used.

Writing in The Medical Journal of Australia, Neil Boyce observed that: "Most current indicators of healthcare performance should be viewed as tools that prompt additional inquiry, rather than allowing definitive judgements on quality and safety of care. They may be defined as norms, criteria, standards, and other direct qualitative and quantitative measures used in determining the quality of care and can therefore be used to judge performance."

Think of an indicator as a torch that shines light on an area of practice that merits further scrutiny. It is the more detailed inquiry prompted by the indicators that will lead to the development of quality measures.

Quality indicators can:
- Allow comparisons to be made between practices and against the gold standard.
- Help to identify unacceptable performance.
- Stimulate informed discussion and debate about the quality of care.
- Facilitate an objective evaluation of a quality improvements initiative.

A good example is the so-called practice visit in the UK. These visits or inspections are undertaken by a number of professional organisations for various purposes ranging from educational bodies that assess a practice's suitability for participating in a postgraduate education programme for recent graduates, to NHS Trusts who often undertake visits when new practices are established in their area. The forms and processes used for these purposes are indicator-driven. When such visits and assessments take place it is important that the results are interpreted in the broader context of the delivery of care rather than making judgements about them.

Quality Measures

Writing in the January 2000 issue of Experience in Practice, Professor John Øvretveit cites the lack of measurement as: "Often the weakest component of a quality programme. Employees often do not have the skills to gather and use quality data, or do not see the need to do so. Professionals do not have the time."

Table 4-1 **Measurements for research and quality improvement**

	Measurement for research	**Measurement for quality improvement**
Purpose	To discover new knowledge	To introduce new knowledge into everyday clinical practice
Tests	Large randomised double-blind clinical trials	Many smaller, sequential, and observable tests
Biases	Methodology is designed to control for as many biases as possible	Stabilise the biases from test to test
Data	Gather as much data as possible, "just in case"	Gather "just enough" data to learn and complete another cycle
Duration	Can take long periods of time to obtain results and for the results to have an impact on clinical practice	"Small tests of significant changes" accelerate the rate of improvement

We should note that:
- No measure is perfect, but together with companion measures, it may still be quite useful.
- Consistency is important. A fundamental concept with measurement is that if we change our method of measuring – our operational definition – we change the data collected.
- If you cannot measure it, then you can't manage it.

Øvretveit states that: "Measurement should speed improvement, not slow it down. Often, organisations get bogged down in measurement, and delay making changes until they have collected all of the data they believe they require. Measurement, *per se*, is not the goal; improvement is the goal." Micromanage and we are likely to lose sight of true purpose.

Quality can be measured in many different ways. The most appropriate measure to use in a given situation is determined by what we are attempting to understand. A measure that is appropriate for one purpose, like measuring the quality of care received by a group of patients under a particular system of remuneration, may not be appropriate for, say, measuring the effectiveness of a clinical guideline.

In general practice, we are likely to use measurements for quality improvement rather than research. This means that the measures need not be as robust or detailed as those required for research. The essential differences are summarised in Table 4-1.

Quality measures can be either quantitative or qualitative. They can be used to look at processes, outcomes and the patient experience.

Quantitative Measures

A quantitative measure provides a quantitative indication of the extent, amount, dimensions, capacity, or size of some attribute of a product or a process.

There are different types of measures summarised in Table 4-2 below:

Binomial Measures
They are most useful for compliance checks or criteria checks – they are often yes/no answers. These are useful for checking the structural elements in a practice, compliance to legislation, and may also be used in some types of audit. The audit example of post sterilisation debris on instruments given in Chapter 6 used a binomial measure for recording the data.

Table 4-2 **Types of measures**

Binomial (i.e. binary)	Like a switch, it either is or isn't. Discrete values such as "0" or "1": "Y[ES]" or "N[O]": "T[RUE]" or "F[ALSE]" are examples of binary values. When stated in terms of a range of values, the value lies within (meets) or outside (exceeds) a threshold
Additive	Simple counts, or rates, of the entity of interest. Best suited for integer-value data
Ratio	The proportion of one value relative to another value
Averages	The mean of a population or sample of data
Statistical	Descriptive and inferential statistics

Additive Measures

Integer-value data are easy to use; consequently they are very popular. They can be used to measure clinical activity – as they will be under local contracting arrangements in the NHS in England and Wales – patient numbers, number of days worked and so on. However, they are sometimes used inappropriately. For example, a practice owner may be concerned about the level of expenditure on dental materials using additive measures to indicate his expenditure over a 12-month period. The data are of no value – a ratio measure would be a better indicator, expressing the information as a percentage of overall turnover, because this would allow for a meaningful comparison against benchmark standards.

Ratio Measures

Ratios are commonly used in everyday life to measure performance. In evaluating a car, we may calculate miles per gallon or the time taken to reach a certain speed as a performance measure. This is a simple ratio of the number of miles driven, divided by the number of gallons of fuel consumed.

They can be used to express many aspects of dental practice – the number of patients seen per week, the proportion of adhesive bridges that may have debonded over a five-year period for example.

Clinical success rates in general practice may be expressed in percentage terms and are examples of a ratio measure – for example, a clinic may claim a 95% success rate in completed root canal treatments over a given period of time.

Other applications in healthcare include the percentage of two-year-old children who receive the appropriate immunisations – this is a simple ratio of the number of two-year-old children with the appropriate immunisations, divided by the total number of two-year-old children in the applicable population. They can also be used to set targets.

Another example may be the percentage of patients reporting that they had no problem in obtaining a specialist referral. Again, this is a simple ratio of the number of patients reporting "no problem" divided by the total number of patients in the applicable population who require a specialist referral. The ratios are often expressed as a percentage. Quality standards can then be set by establishing benchmark ratio measures and may be expressed as percentages.

Ratio measures are also frequently used in clinical audit to compare operator performance against benchmark standards. For example, in an audit of quality of bitewing radiographs the benchmark standard states that not less than 70% of films should be rated "excellent" in relation to defined criteria.

Averages
Patient waiting times for non-urgent appointments is one example.

Statistics
These are used largely in research and are beyond the scope of the present text. Statistics do provide useful information for general practitioners and impact on clinical guidelines and expected standards in clinical practice.

Qualitative Measures

Albert Einstein's observation that "not everything that counts can be counted, and not everything that can be counted counts" emphasises the intrinsic biases and limitations of many data collection measures. To overcome these limitations, we need additional qualitative measures.

Typically, these involve either some form of direct observation of performance, or indirect assessment of performance. Some examples used in dental practice include:
• Observation of service delivery by peers
• Mystery patient method
• Audit of patient records
• Review of data from automated information system
• Peer review
• Patient exit interview
• Patient satisfaction surveys.

Walk-through (IHI Tool)

Dr David Gustafson from the University of Wisconsin describes what he calls a "walk-through tool" – a derivation of management by walkabout. Its purpose is to enable providers to better understand the experience of care from the patient's viewpoint by going through the experience themselves.

Applying Gustafson's principle in general practice has these advantages:
• It provides you with first-hand knowledge of what it is like to be a patient in your practice.
• It builds the will to improve in-practice processes to enhance the patient experience and generate ideas for innovation.
• Direct observations will help to identify feelings such as frustration, anxiety, confidence, and confusion.

Data Gathering

Data gathering and usage is probably the most challenging aspect of measurement. Anecdotal evidence suggests that many dentists fail to find the enthusiasm to undertake such a task, perhaps seeing it as a distraction from the "real work" of treating patients rather than an integral part of practice management. Additionally, we may not have the information management systems for data capture and analysis.

External Evaluation

The external evaluation of quality takes place through:
- Licensing – the formal granting of permission to practise a profession.
- Accreditation – the establishment of the status, legitimacy or appropriateness of an institution or programme of study.
- Certification – the process of formally acknowledging achievement or compliance. It can be used to signify the achievement of an individual, such as a student, or of an institution.
- Revalidation.

Licensing
Established to protect the public, licensing standards address the minimum legal requirements or qualifications to which healthcare professionals and organisations need to conform. Licensing focuses on adherence to minimal standards intended to assure public safety.

Accreditation
Accreditation focuses on continuous improvement strategies, achievement of optimal quality standards, and ongoing education and consultation. It is usually a voluntary process under which an agency grants recognition to healthcare institutions which meet certain standards. The advantages of accreditation are:
- It uses consensus standards.
- It is objective.
- It is proactive not reactive.
- It stimulates a quality culture in the practice.
- It allows for periodic re-evaluation against standards.

For example, the American Academy of Cosmetic Dentistry (AACD) offers its members an accreditation programme outlined in a guide written for the purpose; the American Board of Cosmetic Dentistry is the Credentialing

Authority of the American Academy of Cosmetic Dentistry and its purpose is to test, analyse, and evaluate the services of dentists and laboratory technicians for the purpose of awarding AACD Accreditation in cosmetic dentistry.

Certification

Distinguished from accreditation by its application to both individuals and organisations, certification involves a recognised authority or board granting recognition to individuals who have demonstrated specialised knowledge and skill and to organisations that have the ability to practise in a certain area or specialty.

Revalidation

The aim of revalidation is to enable dental professionals to show that they are up to date and fit to practise. Sir Donald Irvine, President of the General Medical Council between 1995 and 2002, in his book *The doctors' tale: professionalism and public trust* wrote that "Revalidation is based on the positive affirmation of good practice rather than the negative identification of bad apples." The General Dental Council President Hew Mathewson has said that "Compulsory CPD for all our registrants will inform an important component of revalidation." The core subjects for dentists' CPD (continuing professional development) are:

• medical emergencies
• disinfection and decontamination
• radiography and radiation protection.

Collectively, it is recommended that these account for at least 20 hours per CPD cycle; at least 10 hours of medical emergencies and at least 5 hours each for the other areas. Other priority areas for CPD include legal and ethical issues and handling complaints.

Useful Tools

Several tools are available to help with quality measurement because they help with the presentation of data.

Pareto Analysis

The Pareto analysis is a method of classifying items or activities according to their relative importance. It is named after the 19th century Italian economist, Vilfredo Pareto, whose observation that 80% of Italy's wealth was owned by 20% of the population later led to the wider use of what Juran called the 80/20 rule.

The analysis is not scientifically accurate, but a way of identifying what Juran described as "the vital few" issues, and to separate them from "the trivial many". Its purpose is to display data that helps to achieve this separation. Given the limitations of time and resources in a busy practice, tools that assist prioritisation are desirable.

A Pareto chart is a graphical representation that displays data in order of priority (Fig 4-1). The x-axis shows the possible causes and the y-axes represent the frequency and the percentage of the total (right-hand y-axis). It can be a powerful tool for identifying the relative importance of causes, most of which arise from only a few of the processes, hence the 80/20 rule.

Pareto analysis is used to focus problem-solving activities, so that areas creating most of the issues and difficulties are addressed first.

To use this tool in practice, write out a list of the changes you could make. If the list is long, group it into related changes. Then score the items or groups. The scoring method you use depends on the sort of problem you are trying to solve. The first change to tackle is the one that has the highest score. This will deliver the biggest benefit if you are able to solve it.

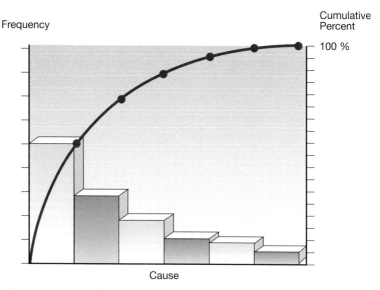

Fig 4-1 Pareto chart.

Example 1

A dentist has concerns about the quality of the service at his practice. A patient survey and various verbal remarks have helped to identify this as an area of concern. These concerns are:

1. The telephone is not answered promptly.
2. Some of the staff seem disorganised and under pressure.
3. Laboratory work is not available on the day of patient appointments and patients have to be rebooked.
4. The compressor is failing and patients have to be rescheduled.
5. Staff members do not always seem to know what they are doing.
6. Records not available at time of appointment.
7. The dentist runs late.

These problems are grouped together and each group is scored by the number of complaints that have been generated by each group.

Punctuality and timekeeping: items 1, 2, 6, 7 – generated 12 complaints.
Poor organisation: item 5, 3 – generated 3 complaints.
Equipment maintenance: item 4 – generated 3 complaints.

By doing a Pareto analysis, we can determine that 12 out of 18 complaints (67%) were the result of poor timekeeping. A root cause analysis would also have identified the same underlying factor. These could be resolved by simply ensuring that team members attend the practice on time, and sufficiently in advance of the first patient to ensure the smooth running of the day.

Example 2

This example shows the use of a Pareto analysis for post-treatment dental emergencies over a four-week period in a dental practice. A post-treatment dental emergency was defined as a patient-led request for an immediate or urgent appointment which was necessary as a direct consequence of recently provided care or treatment. The data is summarised in Table 4-3 overleaf.

The total number of appointments over a four-week period amounted to 21. Of these, 11 related to the communication of post-operative instructions; for example, failing to warn patients about the possibility of pain after root canal therapy, or giving inadequate post-operative instructions. Unscheduled appointments create a disruption in a busy practice and detract from the quality of the patient experience. The outcome of the Pareto analysis would be to ensure that clinicians improved the quality of their communications with patients.

Table 4-3 **Data gathering for a Pareto analysis**

	Complication resulting from the provision of treatment	Post-operative instructions unclear	Patient induced as a result of non-compliance	Other
Week 1	2	3	1	1
Week 2	1	4	0	0
Week 3	2	2	1	0
Week 4	0	2	1	1

Another similar analysis identified that almost 70% of all the unscheduled appointments for one particular clinician in the practice related to post-operative pain following root canal therapy. This was almost double that of other clinicians in the practice and the information could then be used as a basis to review the techniques and processes undertaken by this dentist during root canal treatment.

The analysis can also be used in conjunction with other tools. For example, a clinical audit of the quality of intra-oral radiographs may show that 35% were judged to be unsatisfactory. A Pareto analysis of the unsatisfactory radiographs may highlight processing errors as being responsible for most of the poor-quality images. Attention to this would then bring about significant benefits to the practice and the patients.

In a letter to the British Dental Journal (October 2006), Peter Erridge reflected on his practice management courses in the 1970s, stating that "as a management concept [the Pareto Principle] was introduced to help practitioners to direct their time and effort efficiently".

Client Window
The client window is a tool for gaining feedback from patients. It differs from a patient survey in that a survey asks clients about product or service performance, based on the survey originator's views about what patients want and need. The NHS encourages practitioners to participate in a Patient Forum which is in effect a client window approach.

A client window asks questions in very broad terms. This allows patients to express what they need, expect, like, and dislike in their own words and,

Table 4-4 **The client window template**

	Getting	**Not getting**
Want	Getting what you want	Want, but not getting
Don't want	Getting, but not wanted	Don't want, not getting (anticipated needs for the future)

importantly, from their point of view. It is worth noting that not all things listed will carry equal weight; further discussion will be needed to find which areas are priorities.

To use this tool, first determine the area for which feedback is required. Information can then be gathered by asking the following questions:
• What are you getting that you want?
• What are you getting that is meeting your needs and expectations?
• What are you getting that you really don't want or need?
• What do you wish you were getting that you are not?
• What needs do you expect in the future?
• What suggestions do you have for how we can improve our products or services for you?

A client window can yield the information necessary to conduct more formal data collection through surveys (Table 4-4).

Cause and Effect Diagram
This is known by several different names. It is called the Ishikawa Diagram after the man who invented it, the fishbone diagram after its appearance, or the cause and effect diagram after its use (Fig 4-2). It is often used alongside the technique of root cause analysis.

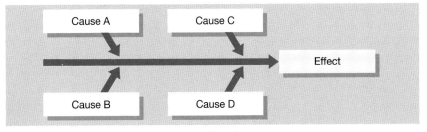

Fig 4-2 Basic layout for a cause and effect diagram.

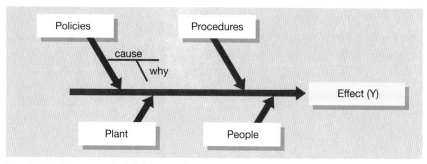

Fig 4-3 The expanded fishbone diagram.

In its basic form, it can be represented as shown in Fig 4-2. The causes can be categorised in various ways (Fig 4-3). The categories used vary depending on the situation and context of use. Examples include:
- materials, methods, machinery operators
- policies, procedures, people, plant.

In a dental practice categories may include:
- product, place, people, price – useful in devising a marketing strategy for the practice
- patient, procedure, materials, technique – this would be suitable for clinical procedures.

To create this type of diagram in your practice:
1. First complete the effect field.
2. Identify the four individual domains relevant to that effect.
3. For each branch identify the factors which may be causes for the effect.
4. For a more detailed diagram, ask the question why when these factors have been identified.

Causes are arranged according to their level of importance and the resulting diagram depicts causal relationships and the associated hierarchy. It is a qualitative tool because of the type of information that is gathered – i.e. words.

The use of a cause and effect tool in general practice is shown in Fig 4-4. It lists the main causes and also some of the sub-causes. A careful analysis of this diagram will identify lack of training in the use of NiTi instruments as the dominant root cause of the adverse outcome.

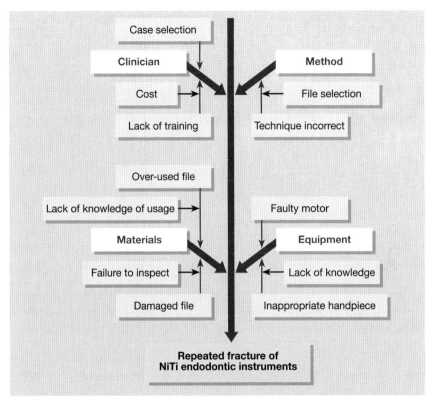

Fig 4-4 Cause and effect diagram to investigate cause of NiTi instrument fracture.

Force Field Analysis

The force field diagram is derived from the work of social psychologist Kurt Lewin who suggested that human behaviour is the result of forces – beliefs, expectations, cultural norms, and so on. These forces can exert a positive influence, urging us toward a behaviour, or a negative influence, propelling us away from a behaviour. It is worth considering the Pareto Principle in relation to this; 80% of the pressure for change or resistance to change will be from 20% of the drivers or resistors to change.

A force field diagram portrays these driving forces and restraining forces that affect a central question or problem. It can be used to compare any kind of opposites, actions and consequences, different points of view, and so on (Fig 4-5).

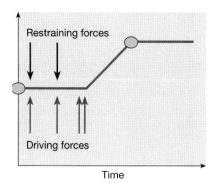

Fig 4-5 Kurt Lewin's Model.

In the context of quality improvement, driving forces could be seen as pushing for change in the practice while restraining forces stand in the way of change. Change occurs only when the driving forces exceed the restraining forces. The most effective way to do this is to diminish (or remove) restraining forces; strengthening the driving forces tends to intensify the opposition at the same time.

Summary

Track only a few key measures over time such as inter-appointment waiting time, new patient consultation times and patient satisfaction. Trends and patterns often emerge and form the basis for any changes. These measures are particularly relevant where third party payers have service level agreements in place, which may define the boundaries for waiting times and the like. Look for practical and pragmatic measures – remember the goal is to improve. Too much data can be stifling for the team and difficult to assimilate.

Sampling by using a random selection of patients is a simple but efficient way to help a team understand how a system is performing. It saves time and resources while accurately tracking performance. Integrate measurement into the daily routine. Useful data are often easy to obtain without relying on information systems.

Use simple data collection forms, and make collecting the data part of someone's job. A few simple measures will yield all the information you need. Use qualitative and quantitative data; qualitative data may be easier to gather and assess and can be highly informative. This can help to develop a hierarchical approach to quality improvement and measurement. It uses a number of essential and desirable indicators, as shown in Table 4-5.

Table 4-5 **A suggested hierarchical model of quality initiatives in general dental practice** (based on a model proposed by Birch, Field and Scrivens[1])

Practice involvement in quality	Some examples of what this might mean
Practice has been externally validated	The practice has completed the national programme but has also achieved additional accreditation through the Fellowship by assessment from the FGDP or Investors in People or ISO 9000
Completion of national programme	The practice has completed a nationally recognised scheme
Active involvement in national programme	The practice is involved in a nationally recognised scheme such as Denplan's Excel programme, BDA's Good Practice Scheme, Smile-on Ltd. clinical governance programme (see Chapter 7) or involvement with Vocational Training
Active involvement in a quality assurance programme	The practice is aware of current issues and adopts a pro-active stance on the quality assurance agenda
Statutory and desirable measures in place	The practice complies with legislation but also has in place some desirable systems of quality assurance over and above the essential requirements
Statutory quality measures all in place	The practice has been visited by the HA and is able to demonstrate compliance with essential legislation
Some quality measures in place	The practice has some elements of essential requirements in place but there are some areas which require attention
Lacking strategic direction	The practice operates on an informal basis with little regard to current trends and has low awareness of current issues.

([1] Birch K, Field S, Scrivens E. Quality in general practice. Radcliffe Medical Press)

One Cautionary Note

You tend to get what you measure for, since people will work to achieve the explicit targets which are set. This behavioural change is an observed phenomenon in many healthcare settings where healthcare workers often meet or exceed set targets for performance.

References

Boyce NW. Potential pitfalls of healthcare performance indicators. Med J Aust 2002;177:229-230.

Erridge P. The Pareto Principle. Letter. Br Dent J 2006;201:419.

Irvine D. The doctors' tale: professionalism and public trust. Oxford: Radcliffe Medical Press, 2003.

Øvretveit J. The Norwegian Approach to Integrated Quality Development. Exp Practice 2000;2.

Further Reading

Koch R. The 80/20 principle: the secret of achieving more with less. New York: Currency Doubleday, 1999.

Chapter 5

Continuous Quality Improvement

Aim

The aim of this chapter is to review the range of options available to practitioners to carry out a quality assessment with a view to embarking on a quality improvement programme.

Outcome

Having read this chapter, the reader should be aware of some of the widely used methods and models that can be used for continuous quality improvement.

Introduction

Quality improvement aims to close the gap between current and expected standards of practice by identifying strengths and weakness in the systems and processes that operate within the practice.

Continuous quality improvement (CQI) theory is important in the general dental practice setting because:
- it gives a rational definition of quality that applies in the healthcare setting
- it clearly shows the relationship between healthcare costs and quality
- it leads to a system under which the highest quality care can consistently be delivered at the lowest justifiable cost.

The range of quality improvement approaches includes:
- problem solving – at individual and team level
- process improvement
- practice redesign and restructuring/reengineering.

These are summarised in Fig 5-1.

Assessment

Before any improvements can be considered, a quality assessment is required, the basic elements of which are summarised in Fig 5-2.

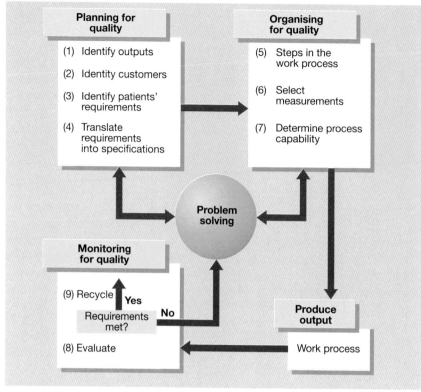

Fig 5-1 The quality improvement process.

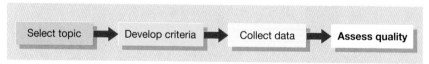

Fig 5-2 Basic elements of a quality assessment.

Topic Selection

The topics to be assessed should be selected based on their significance, feasibility, scope for improvement, and expected results. Selecting a topic on the basis of an adverse outcome is often a good starting point.

Development of Criteria

To be reliable, valid, and reasonable, the chosen criteria must produce similar judgements when assessed by different people. In other words, two people evaluating the same data should draw the same conclusion. For this reason, the criteria must be precise and pertinent to the topic selected and based on supportive evidence; they should be looked upon as a screening device to separate acceptable and unacceptable quality.

Sources of data

Data sources include:

- clinical records
- direct observation of care provision
- patient surveys
- patient interviews.

In practice, we know that each of these data sources has its weaknesses. Incomplete or inadequate clinical records may, for example, give a misleading impression of what was actually done and said. It may be that the provision of clinical care was of a high quality but the actual note taking was inadequate. The idea "if it isn't written down it didn't happen" may be a lawyer's dictum, but it is often not the whole truth. Nevertheless, the dental record is an important data source. At the very least, it should provide a chronological account of the cyclic patient care process, reflecting patient assessment, diagnosis, the treatment plan and execution, and outcome of care.

It is the chronic nature of the most common oral diseases and the repetitive documentation of them that often provides a useful insight into clinical quality. Well structured and properly kept records, together with sequential good quality radiographs, can be a reliable source for data. The use of records is further discussed later in this chapter.

Direct observation is time- and resource-consuming, but is likely to alter the behaviour of those involved in patient-practice interaction. Survey data are known to be inherently subjective and rely on accurate recall of experiences, but are nevertheless useful indicators of the patient experience.

Misconceptions

Improvements in quality are mistakenly taken to mean adding resources. The technological advances in equipment design mean that there is a plethora of gadgets and gizmos to tempt dentists and the assumption has been that adding resources would improve quality, but is this always so? Greater resources do not always ensure their proper and/or efficient use and, consequently, may not lead to improvements in quality. Does the use of Nickel-

Titanium instruments and thermoplastic gutta percha injection techniques improve the clinical outcome in root canal therapy? These may speed up the process of shaping and obturation, and the less aggressive root canal preparation may reduce the risk of root fracture, but the principal determinant in endodontics success remains the efficacy of the irrigation process and the integrity of the coronal seal.

To improve clinical outcomes in endodontics may not necessarily require the structural/resource improvements (per Donabedian's model) based on a purchase, but may simply require an evidence-based approach to root canal irrigation (see Chapter 8). This view is supported in healthcare generally where it has been shown that quality can be improved by making changes to healthcare processes, without necessarily increasing resources.

If, however, an improvement in the process is required, the addition of a resource to achieve the desired outcome would be totally justified; the use of endosonic irrigation in root canal therapy provides an excellent example.

A non-clinical example can be illustrated by one practice's attempt to improve telephone communications with patients. In order to deal with telephone enquiries more efficiently a practice makes an investment in a new telephone system with a call waiting facility. The system is advanced and has many features. Three months after installation, there is no improvement in telephone communications. The reception staff are still unable to cope, and patients have to wait before their calls can be answered. The shortfall in quality is not the telephone system; it is a question of workload management. To improve the telephone service to patients, identify the root cause of the problem and address the processes that lead to the failure (this technique of root cause analysis was discussed more fully in an earlier volume in this series, *Risk Management in General Dental Practice*). The synergy created by first addressing the root cause and *then* adding the resource will bring about a significant improvement in quality.

Approach to Quality Improvement

All approaches to quality improvement rely on some generic principles as summarised in Fig 5-3. One simple but effective four-step process is summarised in Table 5-1. The identification may involve a problem that needs a solution, an opportunity for improvement that requires definition, or a process or system that needs to be improved.

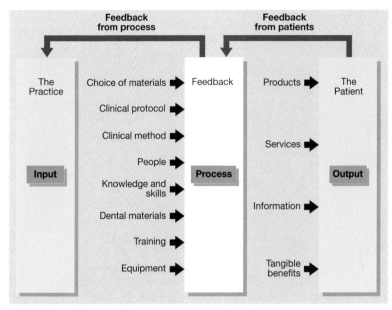

Fig 5-3 Generic elements of quality improvement.

Table 5-1 **A four-step programme for improvement**

1. Identify	**Ask yourself:** What is the problem and how do you know that it is a problem? How frequently does it occur, or how long has it existed? What are the effects of this problem? How will we know when it is resolved?
2. Analyse	**The analysis takes place by asking:** Who is involved or affected? Where does the problem occur? When does the problem occur? What happens when the problem occurs? Why does the problem occur?
3. Develop	This uses the information from the previous stages and explores what improvements may be expected from any planned changes. A strategy for implementing the change is then developed – this will be based on the collective knowledge and experience of the team
4. Test and implement	The final stage tests the effectiveness of the agreed strategy under (3) above to see if the solution produces the desired and anticipated improvements

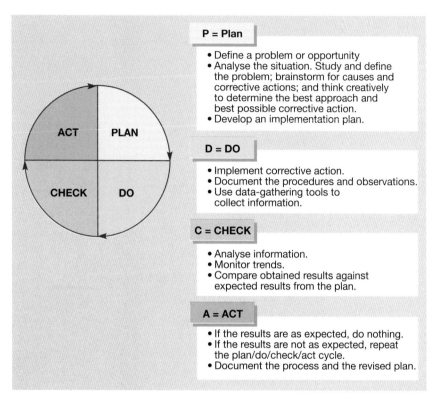

P = Plan
- Define a problem or opportunity
- Analyse the situation. Study and define the problem; brainstorm for causes and corrective actions; and think creatively to determine the best approach and best possible corrective action.
- Develop an implementation plan.

D = DO
- Implement corrective action.
- Document the procedures and observations.
- Use data-gathering tools to collect information.

C = CHECK
- Analyse information.
- Monitor trends.
- Compare obtained results against expected results from the plan.

A = ACT
- If the results are as expected, do nothing.
- If the results are not as expected, repeat the plan/do/check/act cycle.
- Document the process and the revised plan.

Fig 5-4 The PDCA cycle.

The PDCA Cycle

The PDCA cycle was originally conceived by the Bell Laboratories scientist Walter Shewhart in the late 1920s, and further developed by Deming (see Chapter 2). It is shown in Fig 5-4. Applying the cycle continuously leads to what has been described as the ramp of improvement. As each cycle is completed, the next (more advanced and complex) cycle can begin (Fig 5-5).

The word "check" has replaced Deming's original word "study". Shewhart had used the terms "Plan, Do, See".

Ishikawa expanded Deming's PDCA into six segments (Fig 5-6):
- Determine goals and targets.
- Determine methods of reaching goals.

- Engage in education and training.
- Implement work.
- Check the effects of implementation.
- Take appropriate action.

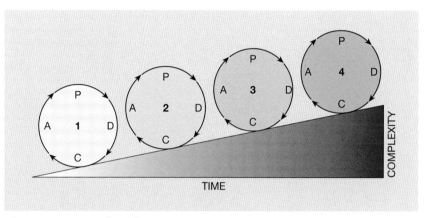

Fig 5-5 Ramping effect of repeated activity using the PDCA cycle.

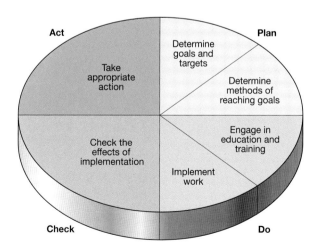

Fig 5-6 The expanded PDCA cycle.
Ishikawa K. (Lu DJ trans.) What is Total Quality Control? Prentice-Hall, 1985.

Limitations

Though widely used, some commentators have highlighted difficulties with this model in the healthcare setting, namely that:

- There is little scientific evidence that CQI improves quality of care.
- There is disparity between the rhetoric and the reality of CQI. The argument is that if we are seeking to create a culture of openness, the threat of external quality assessments, which often accompanies the reality, works against the rhetoric.
- The emphasis on incremental improvements discourages the more radical, discontinuous changes which are sometimes called for.
- The PDCA cycle is better suited to slow-moving industries than to modern, complex, technological settings.

Performance Indicators

Øvretveit defines an indicator as: "A measure that is used to indicate the occurrence of an event where a direct measure cannot be used." Performance indicators are part of an overarching quality framework (Fig 5-7) that seeks to improve patient care and clinical outcomes. Indicators can contribute to quality improvement programmes in two ways: Firstly, they

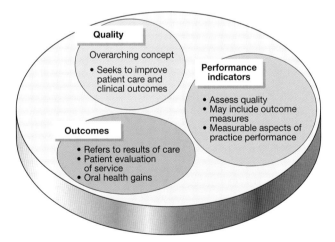

Fig 5-7 Performance indicators as an integral part of quality. Adapted from: Crampton P, Perera R, Crengle S, Dowell A, Howden-Chapman P, Kearns R, Love T, Sibthorpe B, Southwick M. What makes a good performance indicator? Devising primary care performance indicators for New Zealand. Journal of the New Zealand Medical Association;2004(4);Vol.117,No.1191.

can promote wider use of evidence-based interventions; secondly they may assist in the evaluation of quality improvement programmes at a practice level.

Performance indicators assist practices in assessing the effectiveness of their own activities. As there is increasing emphasis on value for money from third party payers, performance indicators are of growing importance. The introduction of local commissioning for primary dental services in England in 2006 coincides with the introduction of the Unit of Dental Activity (UDA) as a performance indicator. The NHS requires the delivery of preset UDA targets for a defined annual budget, but considers re-commissioning of UDAs at a lower cost as added value if a contract is terminated or transferred.

Clinical activity and non-clinical activity which may contribute to the welfare of a patient or contribute to the quality of the patient experience, but which does not qualify for the chosen metric (the UDA) cannot therefore be assessed; this highlights the limitations inherent in this performance indicator.

It demonstrates that the validity, reliability, and acceptability of performance indicators depend to a large extent on their intended uses. The characteristics of useful indicators are summarised in Table 5-2.

What Should Indicators Measure?
In short, indicators should assess quality on the basis of access and effectiveness. In other words, do patients get the care they need, and is the care and treatment effective when they get it? We revert to this in Chapter 8.

Donabedian's model of structure, process and outcome provides a useful reference framework for measurement. From the structure perspective, we can measure elements such as opening hours, practice facilities, the appointment booking system, and the premises. We can also look at human resources such as the skill mix within the dental team.

In terms of outcomes, we should focus on:
• oral health status following care and treatment
• patient satisfaction and experience
• cost (and perceived value)
• equity and fairness.

Table 5-2 **Requirements of useful indicators**

Requirements	Explanation
Reflect important aspects of health status	Example: periodontal disease – the main cause of tooth loss
Be attributable to healthcare	There must be a link between provider actions and the performance indicator that the provider has some control over. Example: clinical intervention and diagnosis
Be linked to health outcomes	There must be evidence that improved indicator values are associated with improved clinical outcomes
Be sensitive to change	Performance indicators should detect changes in provider behaviour
Be based on reliable and valid information	Performance indicators should be evidence-based
Be precisely defined	All parties should work to the same definition
Be easily quantifiable	Numerical presentation is often preferred
Reflect a variety of dimensions of care	Different indicators will be required for different dimensions of care
Be understood by people who need to act	An in-depth knowledge about how and why the indicators were derived is essential
Be relevant to policy and practice	They should serve the needs of providers and commissioners
Be feasible to collect and report	The cost of collecting data for performance indicators should be within the scope of primary care funding
Comply with national definitions	There should be no scope for variation in interpretation
Minimise perverse incentives	Punitive and constructive uses of indicators affect provider behaviour

Adapted from: Crampton P, Perera P, Crengle S, Dowell A, Howden-Chapman P, Kearns R, Love T, Sibthorpe B, Southwick M. What makes a good performance indicator? Devising primary care performance indicators for New Zealand. Journal of the New Zealand Medical Association;2004(4):Vol.117,No. 1191.

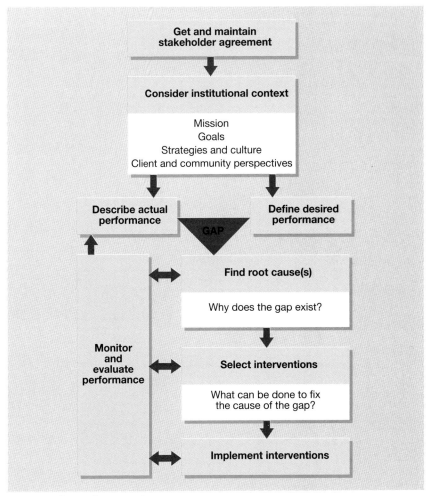

Fig 5-8 The performance improvement process.

Performance Improvement

Performance indicators can help to identify quality gaps and identify areas for improvement (Fig 5-8). In this model, the gap between actual and desired performance is identified and the root cause determined. A useful technique for root cause analysis is the "five-why" technique; ask the question "why" at least five times to determine the root cause of a known quality gap.

Performance review is a feature of many modern healthcare systems. It is often based on the process of peer review, but can also involve other stakeholders. The process is designed to be supportive rather than punitive. Early correction of concerns can often prevent disciplinary action. Those charged with the responsibility of carrying out the review may recommend a range of remedial measures including:

- information sources
- performance support through coaching/mentoring
- appraisal systems
- team building
- formal training and education.

The recommendation should be based on a root cause analysis to ensure that the interventions recommended are based on relevant data and are what is really needed. Often a combination of interventions is implemented as part of a comprehensive solution to address multiple performance factor deficiencies.

An example of such a scheme in the UK is the practitioner advice and support scheme (PASS). One of the earliest such schemes was instigated in Lancashire in 1999 and sets out to:

- facilitate the early identification of dentists whose performance is giving rise to concern
- provide dentists who need access to the scheme with support and guidance to enable them to improve their standards of performance
- assure the public, politicians and the profession that the issue of suboptimal performance is being responsibly addressed.

The concept of PASS is recognised by the General Dental Council (GDC). Advice is provided on how such schemes may be established. Further information can be downloaded from the GDC website: http://www.gdc-uk.org.

Benchmarking

Benchmarking in clinical practice helps to identify standards of excellence and by comparison provides impetus for quality improvement initiatives. The concept is discussed more fully in Chapter 3.

Critical Incidents

Critical incidents create quality improvement opportunities. They are often easy to relate to, and provide real-life scenarios from which everyone can learn.

A critical incident can be any noteworthy event at the practice. It can be a clinical or non-clinical occurrence and may be a positive or negative event. Positive experiences reinforce existing quality improvements processes and negative outcomes can help address shortcomings. Some examples taken from general dental practice include:
- A missed diagnosis necessitating complex intervention – failure to diagnose caries leading to endodontic treatment or extraction
- A prescribing error – issuing penicillin to a patient with a known allergy
- An unexpected medical emergency
- A patient complaint about the practice receptionist
- A staff member resigning unexpectedly due to stress in the workplace
- Clinical records mix-up
- Laboratory work mix-up
- An injury in the workplace
- A thank you letter from a patient
- An award for the practice.

Adverse Events

An adverse event is defined as an accident, incident or occurrence which has:
- resulted in physical or emotional harm to a patient or member of staff – this includes threatening, abusive or violent behaviour
- hindered significantly the effective delivery of services to patients
- damaged the reputation of the practice.

The term "near miss" is used to describe a situation in which an event or omission occurred which could have developed into an adverse incident and caused harm, but didn't. Both provide learning opportunities and should be a catalyst for a quality improvement initiative.

Significant Event Audit

Professor Mike Pringle of Nottingham University describes significant event audit as: "A process of analysis, by those involved, of key events with a view to learning lessons and improving practice."

In a survey carried out by the School of Health and Related Research (ScHARR), the benefits of SEA were identified as:
- making professional practice more satisfying
- greater openness, willingness to learn

- better care for patients
- improvement in professional standards
- improvements in team working
- a shift from an individualistic view of practice to a recognition that practitioners operate in, and are affected by, a wider system.

The process involved in carrying out SEA is summarised in Table 5-3.

When the review has been completed, a record should be kept. These records can be reviewed over a period of time to see if there are any emerging trends or patterns.

The risk consulting arm of the Medical Protection Society states that if run properly, SEA should be voluntary, blame-free, supportive, reflective, educational, internal to the practice, confidential, and a celebration of good practice in the case of positive incidents. It should also:
- Highlight areas for attention
- Minimise risk within the practice
- Encourage excellence.

Table 5-3 **How to conduct SEA**

Identify and record the incident	Prepare the review	Run the review
Describe what happened How did it affect the patient? How did it affect you? How did it affect the practice? How could it have been avoided? What opportunities are there for learning as a result of this?	Somebody should lead the review and it should be carried out in an open and blame-free manner with ample opportunities for all to speak and listen. Confidentiality is important and must be assured.	The questions shown in the first column provide a route map for the review.

Using Clinical Records

Comprehensive clinical records do not ensure the adequacy of dental care, just as incomplete records do not infer that the quality of care and treatment is poor. However, if well maintained, clinical records can be very useful in quality assessment.

According to Marshall (1996): "The most important tool in dental quality assurance is the patient record, when properly structured and maintained. It is the only instrument that is capable of documenting all aspects of patient care that can readily be used to gain insight into not only the clinician's adequacy in diagnosis and treatment planning, but also into the sequencing of treatment procedures, their delivery and, in conjunction with radiographs, the technical quality of the procedures themselves."

There are limitations to the value of the clinical record; for example, it cannot help to determine aesthetics, accuracy of fit of fixed and removable prostheses and occlusal relationships, unless supporting statements (and photographs), based on explicit criteria, can provide this level of detail. A statement that reads "good fit" is subjective unless "goodness" is defined by objective criteria. That is not to say that subjective statements are not helpful. A comment like "patient pleased with appearance" would be a reliable patient satisfaction indicator and, as such, can contribute to a user-defined definition of quality.

Peer review by a means of direct examination of the patient is an option, but has been discarded for reasons of expense, and is unacceptable to many practitioners. Random and targeted examinations of some patients are a feature of many third party payment systems. The NHS in the UK uses a process which involves dental reference officers who examine patients and report on their oral health status – and share their findings in reports to the third party payer and the dentist.

Summary

Quality improvement principles apply to technical quality, as evaluated primarily by clinicians and to the delivery, as evaluated primarily by patients.

Reference

Marshall KF. Evaluating quality through records and radiographs: a rationale for general dental practice. Br Dent J 1996;179:234-235.

Chapter 6
Clinical Audit

Aims

This chapter aims to explain the principles of clinical audit and how the process of clinical audit can be used as a quality improvement tool. It also aims to give examples of audits where there has been a demonstrable improvement in performance as a result of carrying out the audit.

Outcome

Having read this chapter, the reader should be aware of the importance of clinical audit as a quality improvement tool and understand how the principles of audit may be applied to clinical practice.

Introduction

Clinical audit is an important quality improvement process, and a most effective tool for clinical governance. In the UK, the Department of Health described clinical audit (and peer review) as "a central pillar of clinical governance" and all dentists practising within the NHS were required to participate in a rolling programme of audits/peer reviews. This improvement in quality will be reflected in:
- improved care of patients
- consistent care of patients
- enhanced professionalism of staff
- efficient use of resources
- more effective administration
- accountability to those outside the profession
- increased patient satisfaction.

It is not a new process; as early as 1750 BC, King Hammurabi of Babylon involved clinicians in audit, with financial penalties being imposed in the event of poor performance.

Audit has been defined in the UK by both the National Institute for Health and Clinical Excellence (NICE) and the Healthcare Commission as: "A quality improvement process that seeks to improve the patient care and outcomes through systematic review of care against explicit criteria and the implementation of change. Aspects of the structures, processes and outcomes of care are selected and systematically evaluated against explicit criteria. Where indicated, changes are implemented at an individual, team, or service level and further monitoring is used to confirm improvement in healthcare delivery."

Audits can take a retrospective or prospective sample. Retrospective audit looks at past care. It is particularly useful where there has been a critical incident such as a patient complaint, adverse outcome or litigation. Such incidents usually prompt an urgent review of processes and standards and audit provides the mechanism.

Prospective audit looks at future care. Unlike retrospective audit, it reflects current practice and allows for accurate real time accrual of data, which means that the data should be accurate both in terms of detail and volume.

The Audit Cycle

Clinical audit is often described as a cycle or a spiral (Fig 6-1).

Selecting an Audit Project
An audit project may be selected on the basis of:
- high volume
- high risk
- high profile
- high cost
- known weaknesses.

We should ask the following questions:
- Is there any evidence of a serious quality problem?
  Are there patient complaints or high post-operative patient return/complication rates?
- Is good evidence available to inform standards?
  Standards will need to be identified – we need to know where we can source these.
- Is the identified problem amenable to change?
  If there is limited scope for change, then the value of the audit is limited because it may not be possible to achieve sustainable improvement.
- Why is the topic a priority for the practice?
  Why should this topic be selected above others?

- Will team members recognise the value of the audit?
  The team must recognise the importance and the value of the topic. Team buy-in is important to implement effective change.

Undertaking the Audit

To undertake the audit, we need to address the following questions:
- Will the data be collected retrospectively or prospectively?
- What is the sample size?
- What are the sample criteria to be?
- What data do you want to collect?
- Who will collect the data?
- Who will analyse the data?
- How will data be collected, i.e. using a computer or by hand?

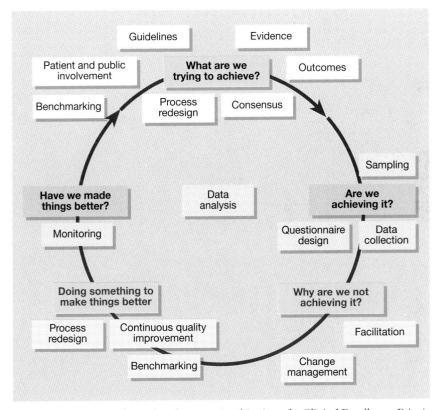

Fig 6-1 The audit cycle. Taken from: National Institute for Clinical Excellence. Principles for best practice in clinical audit. Oxford: Radcliffe Medical Press, 2002.

Review the Findings

Having collected and analysed your data, you will need to identify what areas may need changing. This can be done by:

- summarising your findings in a form that is easy to digest
- arranging a team meeting to discuss the audit results
- adopting an agreed strategy for change.

Implementation of Change

Having decided what changes are needed, you will have to consider a reasonable time frame in which to implement the changes. This means:

- agreeing on a date to re-audit
- producing an audit report
- ways to share your findings if applicable.

Repeating the Cycle

Audit is a continuous cycle – this is why the term audit spiral is a more appropriate one. If the standard has not been met and changes have been planned, the audit will need to be repeated to ensure that the changes have happened. It is important to close this loop and re-evaluate the situation to ensure that any remedial action has been effective.

Example

In a prospective waiting times audit carried out in general practice, the data was collected using a commercially available clinical audit CD ROM which used Microsoft Excel spreadsheets to record, process and present the data in an easy-to-understand format. The pre- and post-audit results are shown in Fig 6-2. This topic was selected as a result of patient complaints. Changes were made to the appointment control system as a result of the initial audit, with contributions from members of the team.

An audit report was prepared and the data presented in graphics. Four weeks later, a further audit was undertaken. The re-audit data shows the improvements that were achieved.

Standards

Standards are integral to clinical audit; they can be clinical or managerial and can be applied at individual or at practice level. They communicate an expectation of clinical or non-clinical performance for both dentists and patients and what is needed to provide a quality service.

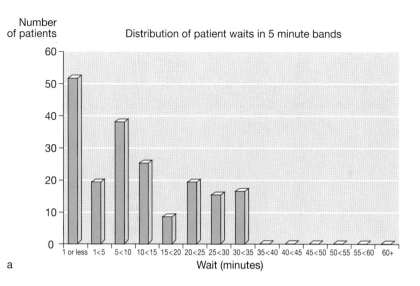

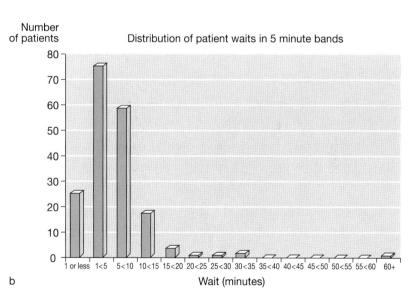

Fig 6-2 (a,b) (a) Initial data of an audit of patient waiting times. (b) Re-audit data after changes.

A standard is an explicit statement of expected quality in the performance of a given clinical or non-clinical activity. Performance in accordance with standards is thus the cornerstone of quality assurance in everyday practice because adherence to evidence-based standards is associated with improved clinical outcomes. Failure to provide clinical care to explicit standards has serious negative effects on patient outcomes.

A standards-based approach to quality is not new. Juran noted that the Zhou dynasty of China (around 1000 BC) decreed: "Utensils under standard are not allowed to be sold on the market; carts under standard are not allowed to be sold on the market; cottons and silk of which the quality and size are not up to standard are not allowed to be sold on the market."

More recently, The Bristol Royal Infirmary Inquiry (2001) in the UK reported that: "Central to the concept of audit is the idea that standards of clinical care should first be set; then performance assessed, and possible improvements in practice identified and implemented."

Standards may be developed by government health agencies, professional bodies, specialist societies, international organisations (e.g. the World Health Organization), professional accrediting organisations and also by the process of peer review. The latter is particularly important when it comes to auditing aspects of practice where the reference material for standards may be lacking. The accepted standard for waiting times in the example quoted earlier in this chapter was established in this way.

Standards are often described as explicit (written), or implicit (understood). Implicit standards are derived from the collective expertise of the profession. By converting implicit standards to explicit standards, we can reduce variations in treatment planning and execution amongst dentists, and provide a baseline measure for monitoring quality.

Explicit standards appear in a variety of forms, such as procedures, protocols, or clinical practice guidelines (Table 6-1).

Clinical practice guidelines have been developed primarily by clinicians to guide their practice, whereas protocols and procedures are designed for more general use, often with input from professional associations.

Table 6-1 **Standard formats and usage**

Format	Description	Use
Clinical practice guidelines	Recommendations for dental care based on current research	For reference by dentists for management of specific situations or conditions
Clinical pathways	Expected, multidisciplinary plan of treatment – primarily used in hospitals at present	By the professional team to plan the progress of care
Algorithms	Flowcharts or decision grid	Very visual – help to make quick decisions
Procedures	How to type instructions	Directions on how to perform a technical skill, e.g. impression taking
Protocols	Management of patient care	Patient care management for specific situations, e.g. a patient with a specific medical condition

If they are to be widely adopted and respected, standards must be:
- Explicit – written, clear and easily understood.
- Realistic – the standards can be followed or achieved with existing resources.
- Reliable – if a dentist follows a guideline for a specific intervention, then the outcome should be the same each time provided there are no other variables.
- Valid – the standards should derive from an evidence-based approach.
- Clear – they should not be subject to misinterpretation.
- Measurable – it should be possible to assess performance against the standard.

What Makes an Audit a Useful Audit?

The characteristics of useful and useless audits are summarised in Table 6-2.

Table 6-2 **Useful vs. useless audits**

Characteristics of a "useful" audit	Characteristics of a "useless" audit
• That practices examine areas of care that need to be examined • Standards which are set relate to local and national standards. If there are none, that the practice sets its own realistic standards or consults with peers to set peer reference standards • There is team involvement. Audit is almost always a team effort • Analysis of the collected data takes place and is compared to set standards • Changes are realistic, acceptable, and bring demonstrable benefits to the practice and the patients • There is evidence of change • That re-audit happens to enable comparisons with previous results	• Topic chosen has no relevance to practice needs – it may be one person's pet topic which has little relevance or importance to other members of the team • Topic that no one wants to take on, because they have not been involved or because it has been imposed • Standards are non-existent, or too high or too low • Poor methodology, poor data collection, and too large or too small a sample • Analysis is inadequate or not meaningful • There is no comparison to the set standards • No changes are made and if made there is no ownership of change

Examples

Pessian and Beckett undertook an audit of the quality of record cards amongst undergraduate dental students. Their reason for selecting the topic was based on earlier studies which showed the quality of dental records to be generally "poor". Their view of the importance of clinical records accords with that cited in other parts of this text, namely that: "Although good records do not ensure the adequacy of dental care, they do provide an opportunity to evaluate it, which poor records do not. Therefore for a quality assurance programme to be fully effective, the clinical records must be maintained at a level that allows proper assessment of care provided."

Using criteria established by the UK Faculty of General Dental Practitioners, they reviewed 100 records and noted some improvements in the standard of record keeping after students received a tutorial on the subject following the first audit. The results relating to the "medical history" and "patient complaint" components showed deterioration however. The audit and re-audit results are shown in Fig 6-3.

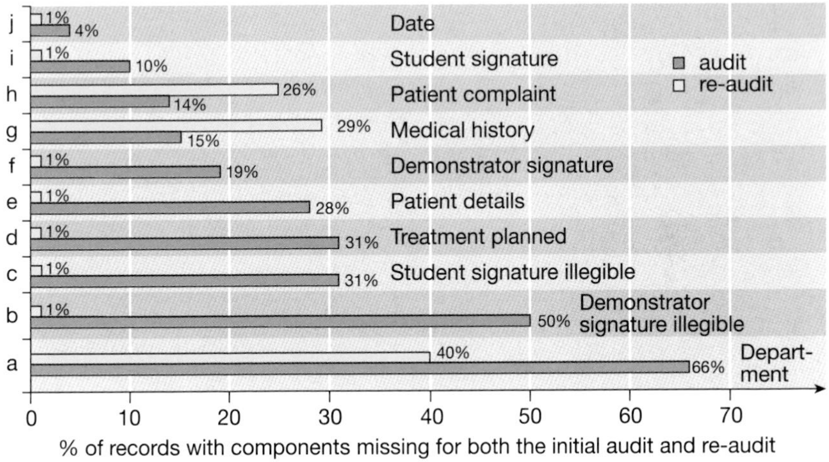

Fig 6-3 Audit results on record keeping involving students.

Another study by Palmer, Dailey and Martin (2001) looked at the changes in prescribing habits of dentists. The results of a pre- and post-audit of the prescribing activity of dentists are shown in Fig 6-4. This audit showed that: "Using guidelines, and an educational component with feedback, was effective in reducing inappropriate antimicrobial use by changing GDPs' prescribing practices."

Another good example of an audit which would be useful in practice was one that looked at the extent of debris remaining on post sterilisation instruments which resulted in rejection of use.

This practice-based investigation carried out by the NHS Education for Scotland (NES) involved random selections of instruments – in groups of 10 instruments – from the five types most likely to be contaminated in each of the four surgeries in one practice.

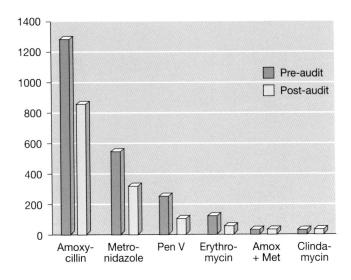

Fig 6-4 Antibiotic audit results.

This was done prior to additional training or encouragement in the use of ultrasonic baths. This identified a baseline of rejection to allow assessment of future training/practice changes.

The process was carried out without the staff knowing what was being checked. The criterion used was one of zero tolerance of debris – most deposits found were very small. The instruments were either recorded as:
1. acceptable, no debris visible
2. rejected, debris visible.

The baseline recorded a 37% rejection rate, but this had dropped to 10% after further in-practice training had been implemented (Fig 6-5).

These examples demonstrate that clinical audit is an effective tool for quality improvement in clinical practice.

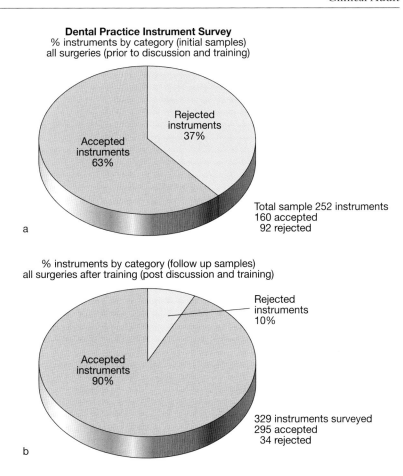

Figs 6-5 (a,b) (a) The baseline audit (b) Re-audit results after training.

References

Faculty of General Dental Practice (UK). Clinical Examination and Record Keeping: Good Practice Guidelines. London: FGDP, 2001.

Palmer NA, Dailey YM, Martin MV. Can audit improve antibiotic prescribing in general dental practice? Br Dent J 2001;191:253-235.

Pessian F, Beckett HA. Record keeping by undergraduate dental students: a clinical audit. Br Dent J 2004;197:703-705.

Chapter 7
Clinical Governance

Aims

This chapter aims to explain the meaning and interpretation of clinical governance and to illustrate how the Healthcare Commission's framework can be applied to general dental practice.

Outcome

After reading this chapter, the reader should be familiar with the principles and application of clinical governance in everyday practice.

Introduction

In England and Wales, Clinical Governance (CG) is the vehicle for the delivery of quality healthcare in the NHS. The Labour government introduced the concept in 1999 in the white paper *The New NHS: Modern, Dependable.* It came about as a result of various NHS scandals through the 1990s, but concerns were expressed about the purpose and process.

David Haslam, a general practitioner and respected writer, noted that:
"The concept of clinical governance has become something as unwelcome as a dental check-up. We know that we have to do it; we know that it is really for the best, but we simply cannot dig deep and find any enthusiasm for the process."

Neville Goodman, a consultant anaesthetist in Bristol, wrote that *"the most important elements in the delivery of quality in healthcare are contained in the relations between human beings. With good working relationships clinical governance happens naturally; with poor working relations, setting up committees and defining quality on bits of paper delivers only bits of paper."*

A duty of quality was placed on NHS organisations in the 1999 NHS Act. In Section 18(1) it states that: *"It is the duty of each Health Authority, Primary Care Trust and NHS Trust to put and keep in place arrangements for the purpose of monitoring and improving the quality of health care which it provides to individuals."*

93

This Act introduced corporate accountability for clinical quality and performance. Clinical Governance is described as a *"whole system"* process with the following features:

- Patient-centred care needs are at the heart of every NHS organisation. This means that patients are kept well informed and are given the opportunity to participate in their care.
- Good information about the quality of services is available to those providing the services as well as to patients and the public.
- Variations in the process, outcomes and in access to healthcare are greatly reduced.
- NHS organisations and partners work together to provide quality assured services and drive forward continuous improvement.
- Health professionals work in teams to a consistently high standard and identify ways to provide safer and even better care for their patients.
- Risks and hazards to patients are reduced to as low a level as possible, creating a safety culture throughout the NHS.
- Good practice and research evidence is systematically adopted.

Consequently, in 2001, it became a requirement for dentists practising in the NHS to have a quality assurance system in place. The new dental contract in 2006 places further emphasis on this requirement.

The Health and Social Care (Community Health and Standards) Act 2003 refers to the "duty of quality" and states that it is the duty of each NHS body to put and keep in place arrangements for the purpose of monitoring and improving the quality of healthcare provided by and for that body.

Definition

Clinical Governance is a system through which NHS organisations are accountable for continuously improving the quality of their services and safeguarding high standards of care by creating an environment in which excellence in clinical care will flourish. (Scally and Donaldson) (Fig 7-1)

Roy Lilley, a prolific writer on healthcare matters, took the view that it was about *"doing anything and everything required to maximise quality"*.

Adding the words *"by everyone"* makes it an inclusive activity involving all members of the dental team.

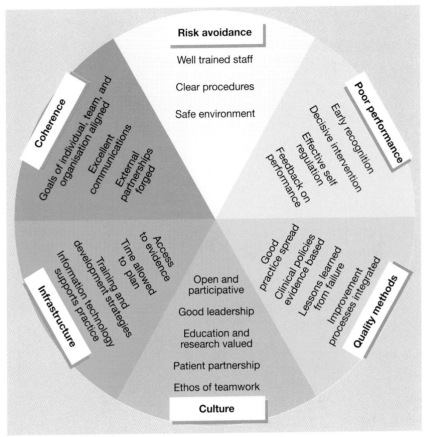

Fig 7-1 Approaches to clinical governance.
From: Scally G, Donaldson, L. Looking forward: Clinical governance and the drive for quality improvement in the new NHS in England. BMJ 1998;317(7150):61-65.

The Royal College of General Practitioners defines it in relation to activities by describing it as *"a framework for the improvement of patient care through commitment to high standards, reflective practice, risk management, and personal and team development."*

The underlying ten principles of CG were first set out in *The New NHS: Modern, Dependable.* These are:

1. Evidence-based practice
2. The dissemination of good ideas in practice
3. Quality improvement processes
4. Use of high quality data to monitor clinical care
5. Clinical risk reduction programmes
6. Investigation of adverse events
7. Learning from complaints
8. Dealing with poor performance
9. Implementation of professional development programmes
10. Leadership skill development.

In this publication, the Department of Health has clearly stated the importance of quality control in the NHS by stating that:
"Every part of the NHS and everyone who works in it should take responsibility for working to improve quality. This must be quality in the broadest sense; doing the right thing at the right time for the right people and doing them right first time. And it must be quality of the patient's experience as well as the clinical result-quality measured in terms of prompt access, good relationships and efficient administration."

Aims

CG sets out to ensure that:
- systems to monitor the quality of clinical practice are in place and are functioning properly
- clinical practice is reviewed and improved as a result
- practitioners meet standards, such as those issued by the national professional regulatory bodies
- practitioners adhere to best practice guidelines.

The idea is to raise standards generally which means pushing the profession's whole performance profile up. As dentists recognise something as good practice, and define it as a guideline, so more dentists will adopt the practice, thereby shifting the mean standards of practice (Fig 7-2).

Government Agencies

As part of its drive for quality in healthcare, the British Government has created a number of organisations (Table 7-1). The work and remit of these agencies affects dental practice; their involvement is likely to be strengthened from 2006 with the advent of local contracting and commissioning. The characteristics of these are summarised in Table 7-1 (pages 98-99).

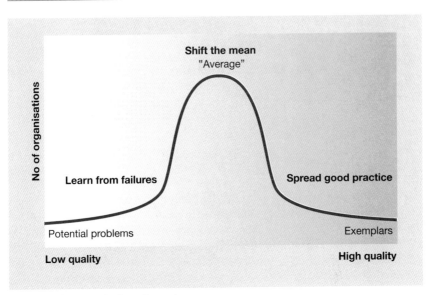

Fig 7-2 The spread of good practice.

National Patient Safety Agency (NPSA)

The NPSA is a Special Health Authority created in July 2001 to coordinate the efforts of the entire country to report, and more importantly to learn from mistakes and problems that affect patient safety. It encourages all health-care staff to report incidents without undue fear of personal reprimand and has recently launched its publication *Medical Error* to redouble its efforts in this respect.

Examples of its advisory work relevant to dentistry include the information published in May 2005 on how to better protect patients with latex allergy. This is available from the NPSA website.

NICE

The National Institute for Health and Clinical Excellence is a special health authority for England and Wales. Its role is to provide patients and health professionals with "authoritative, robust and reliable guidance on current 'best practice'."

Table 7-1 Characteristics of the four NHS regulators created by the British Government

Name	Who it regulates	Date est.	Mission or purpose	How it works	What it is
National Institute for Health and Clinical Excellence (www.nice.org.uk)	NHS in England and Wales	April 1999	To provide patients, health professionals, and the public with authoritative, robust, and reliable guidance on current "best practice"	Uses teams of experts to review health technologies and interventions and produce guidance which is then disseminated	A special health authority, set up by statutory instrument (SI 1999 Nos 220 and 2219)
Commission for Healthcare Audit and Inspection (Healthcare Commission) (www.healthcarecommission.org.uk)	NHS in England and Wales	Nov. 1999	To help improve the quality of patient care by assisting the NHS in addressing unacceptable variations and to ensure a consistently high standard of patient care	Undertakes clinical governance reviews of all NHS organisations every 4 years; monitors implementation of guidelines from NICE, national service frameworks, etc; investigates major system failures within the NHS	A non-departmental public body established by the Health Act 1999

National Patient Safety Agency (www.npsa. org.uk)	NHS in England (at present)	July 2001	To collect and analyse information on adverse events in the NHS, assimilate safety information from elsewhere, learn lessons and feed back to the NHS, produce solutions, set national goals and establish mechanisms to track progress	Operates a new, mandatory national system for reporting adverse events and "near misses," and provides national leadership and guidance on patient safety and adverse events	A special health authority set up by statutory instrument (SI 2001 No 1743)
National Clinical Assessment Service (www.ncaa. nhs.uk)	NHS in England (at present)	April 2001	To provide a support service to health authorities and hospital and community trusts who are faced with concerns over the performance of an individual doctor/dentist	Deals with concerns about doctors in difficulty by providing advice, taking referrals and carrying out targeted assessments where necessary	A special health authority set up by statutory instrument (SI 2000 No 2961). In April 2005, it became part of the NPSA.

NICE guidance covers three areas:
1. Clinical guidelines – these cover the appropriate treatment and care of patients with specific diseases and conditions within the NHS in England and Wales.
2. Technology appraisals cover the use of new treatments within the NHS in England and Wales.
3. Interventional procedures cover the safety and efficacy of interventional procedures for diagnosis and treatment.

The publications relevant to dentistry are:
• Guidance on removal of third molars
• Dental recall (clinical guideline 19 published in October 2004)
• Use of HealOzone in the treatment of pit and fissure caries and root caries (technology appraisal 92, July 2005).

It is now a requirement under clause 71 of the General Dental Services Contract for dentists working in the NHS to apply the NICE guidance when advising patients of the recall interval between their clinical examinations. To assist with this process, NICE has drawn up a clinical risk assessment framework, shown in Table 7-2 (pages 102-103).

It is an expectation within the clinical governance framework that dentists adopt a risk-based approach to setting an appropriate recall interval for their patients.

The Healthcare Commission

The Healthcare Commission (HC) is the name of the independent inspectorate body for the NHS in England; the legal name of the HC is the "Commission for Healthcare Audit and Inspection".

It was formed by the Health and Social Care (Community Health and Standards) Act 2003, and launched on April 1st 2004. It replaces and takes over the functions of a number of regulators of the NHS including its predecessor the Commission for Health Improvement (CHI). Its range of responsibilities is aimed at improving the quality of healthcare. It has a statutory duty to:
• assess the management, provision and quality of NHS healthcare and public health services
• review the performance of each NHS trust
• regulate the independent healthcare sector through registration, annual inspection, monitoring complaints and enforcement

- publish information about the state of healthcare
- consider complaints about NHS organisations that the organisations themselves have not resolved
- promote the coordination of reviews and assessments carried out by itself and others
- carry out investigations of serious failures in the provision of healthcare.

In carrying out its duties, the HC is required to pay particular attention to:
- the availability of, access to, quality and effectiveness of healthcare
- the economy and efficiency of the provision of healthcare
- the availability and quality of information provided to the public about healthcare
- the need to safeguard and promote the rights and welfare of children and the effectiveness of measures taken to do so.

It should be emphasised that the powers of the Commission extend beyond the NHS and include the independent (non NHS) sector. It will regulate independent dentists who provide listed services, as described in the Private and Voluntary Healthcare Regulations (England) 2001. Listed services include class 3b (except where such treatment is carried out by, or under the supervision of, a healthcare professional), class 4 lasers and intense pulsed light sources.

The Commission urges *"unregistered dentists who currently provide these services to make application for registration to the Healthcare Commission without delay. It is an offence under section 11(i) of the Care Standards Act 2000 to carry on or manage an establishment that provides registerable services without being registered. Continuing to provide such services may lead to prosecution."*

The General Dental Services' Contractual Requirements

The standard General Dental Services contract issued in 2006 sets out the requirements for quality assurance in Part 16 (see Table 7-3, page 104).

Interestingly, the original draft of the contract which was published in December 2005, contained the word *"cooperate"* in clause 245 and this was later substituted with the word *"comply"* in a contract variation notice that was issued to dentists on 13 March 2006 – clear indication of the absolute requirement for clinical governance.

Table 7-2 **NICE risk assessment** (continued over page)

Oral health review date:

	Yes	No	Yes	No	Yes	No
Medical history						
Conditions where dental disease could put the patient's general health at increased risk (such as cardiovascular disease, bleeding disorders, immunosuppression)	☐	☐	☐	☐	☐	☐
Conditions that increase a patient's risk of developing dental disease (such as diabetes, xerostomia)	☐	☐	☐	☐	☐	☐
Conditions that may complicate dental treatment or the patient's ability to maintain their oral health (such as special needs, anxious/nervous/phobic conditions)	☐	☐	☐	☐	☐	☐
Social history						
High caries in mother and siblings	☐	☐	☐	☐	☐	☐
Tobacco use	☐	☐	☐	☐	☐	☐
Excessive alcohol use	☐	☐	☐	☐	☐	☐
Family history of chronic or aggressive (early onset/juvenile) periodontitis	☐	☐	☐	☐	☐	☐
Dietary habits						
High and/or frequent sugar intake	☐	☐	☐	☐	☐	☐
High and/or frequent dietary acid intake	☐	☐	☐	☐	☐	☐
Exposure to fluoride						
Use of fluoride toothpaste	☐	☐	☐	☐	☐	☐
Other sources of fluoride (for example, lives in a water-fluoridated area)	☐	☐	☐	☐	☐	☐
Clinical evidence and dental history						
Recent and previous caries experience						
New lesions since last check-up	☐	☐	☐	☐	☐	☐
Anterior caries or restorations	☐	☐	☐	☐	☐	☐
Premature extractions because of caries	☐	☐	☐	☐	☐	☐
Past root caries or large number of exposed roots	☐	☐	☐	☐	☐	☐
Heavily restored dentition	☐	☐	☐	☐	☐	☐

Table 7-2 **NICE risk assessment** (continued)

Oral health review date:						
	Yes	No	Yes	No	Yes	No
Recent and previous periodontal disease experience						
Previous history of periodontal disease	☐	☐	☐	☐	☐	☐
Evidence of gingivitis	☐	☐	☐	☐	☐	☐
Presence of periodontal pockets (BPE code 3 or 4) and/or bleeding on probing	☐	☐	☐	☐	☐	☐
Presence of furcation involvements or advanced attachment loss (BPE code★; that is, attachment loss is at least 7mm and/or furcation involvements are present)	☐	☐	☐	☐	☐	☐
Mucosal lesions						
Mucosal lesion present	☐	☐	☐	☐	☐	☐
Plaque						
Poor level of oral hygiene	☐	☐	☐	☐	☐	☐
Plaque-retaining factors (such as orthodontic appliances)	☐	☐	☐	☐	☐	☐
Saliva						
Low saliva flow rate	☐	☐	☐	☐	☐	☐
Erosion and tooth surface loss						
Clinical evidence of tooth wear	☐	☐	☐	☐	☐	☐
Recommended recall interval for next oral health review:	months		months		months	
Does patient agree with recommended interval?	Yes	No	Yes	No	Yes	No
If "No" record reason for disagreement in notes overleaf						

Shaded boxes represent factors that may increase a patient's risk of or from oral disease.

Table 7-3 **The GDS contractual requirements for quality**

Part 16 Clinical governance and quality assurance

Clinical governance arrangements

245   The Contractor shall comply with such *clinical governance arrangements* as the PCT may establish in respect of contractors providing services under a general dental services contract.

246   The Contractor shall nominate a person who –

246.1   will have responsibility for ensuring compliance with *clinical governance arrangements*; and

246.2   performs or manages services under the Contract.

Quality assurance system

247   The Contractor shall establish, and operate a practice based quality assurance system which is applicable to all persons specified.

248   The specified persons are –

248.1   any dental practitioner who performs services under the Contract; and

248.2   any other person employed or engaged by the Contractor to perform or assist in the performance of services under the Contract.

249   The Contractor shall ensure that in respect of its practice based quality assurance system, it has nominated a person (who need not be connected with the Contractor's *practice*) to be responsible for operating that system.

250   A "practice based quality assurance system" means one which comprises a system to ensure that –

250.1   effective measures of infection control are used;

250.2   all legal requirements relating to health and safety in the workplace are satisfied;

250.3   all legal requirements relating to radiological protection are satisfied;

250.4   any requirements of the General Dental Council in respect of the continuing professional development of dental practitioners are satisfied; and

250.5   the requirement to display in a prominent position the written statement relating to the quality assurance system is satisfied.

The framework referred to in clause 245 used by Primary Care Trusts (PCTs) is that put forward by the Healthcare Commission.

The Healthcare Commission's Framework

As of April 2005, the approach of the HC to quality assurance and standards setting has been to create a framework that is common to all of healthcare – one framework to be populated with criteria and guidance specific to each branch of healthcare. Driven by the publication *Standards for Better Health*, which sets out the level of quality all organisations providing NHS care will be expected to meet or aspire to across the NHS in England, it puts quality firmly at the forefront of the agenda for the NHS.

Expressed as core and development standards, the focus is on providing a common set of requirements applying across all healthcare organisations to ensure the provision of health services that are both safe and of an acceptable quality; there is also emphasis on the process of continuous quality improvement.

The standards describe the level of quality that healthcare organisations, including dental practices, will be expected to meet. There are 24 core standards (one does not apply to general dental practice) and 13 developmental standards prefixed with the letters C and D to indicate their status. The standards are organised into 7 domains. There is an outcome statement (inspired by Donabedian's approach – see Chapter 3) for each domain. These are summarised below.

First Domain – Safety

Domain Outcome
Patient safety is enhanced by the use of health care processes, working practices and systemic activities that prevent or reduce the risk of harm to patients.

Core Standards
C1
Health care organisations protect patients through systems that
a) identify and learn from all patient safety incidents and other reportable incidents, and make improvements in practice based on local and national experience and information derived from the analysis of incidents; and
b) ensure that patient safety notices, alerts and other communications concerning patient safety which require action are acted upon within required timescales.

C2
Health care organisations protect children by following national child protection guidance within their own activities and in their dealings with other organisations.

C3
Health care organisations protect patients by following NICE Interventional Procedures guidance.

C4
Health care organisations keep patients, staff and visitors safe by having systems to ensure that
a) the risk of health care acquired infection to patients is reduced, with particular emphasis on high standards of hygiene and cleanliness, achieving year-on-year reductions in MRSA;
b) all risks associated with the acquisition and use of medical devices are minimised;
c) all reusable medical devices are properly decontaminated prior to use and that the risks associated with decontamination facilities and processes are well managed;
d) medicines are handled safely and securely; and
e) the prevention, segregation, handling, transport and disposal of waste is properly managed so as to minimise the risks to the health and safety of staff, patients, the public and the safety of the environment.

Developmental Standard
D1
Health care organisations continuously and systematically review and improve all aspects of their activities that directly affect patient safety and apply best practice in assessing and managing risks to patients, staff and others, particularly when patients move from the care of one organisation to another.

Second Domain – Clinical and Cost Effectiveness
Domain Outcome
Patients achieve health care benefits that meet their individual needs through health care decisions and services based on what assessed research evidence has shown provides effective clinical outcomes.

Core Standards
C5
Health care organisations ensure that
a) they conform to NICE technology appraisals and, where it is available, take into account nationally agreed guidance when planning and delivering treatment and care;
b) clinical care and treatment are carried out under supervision and leadership;
c) clinicians continuously update skills and techniques relevant to their clinical work; and
d) clinicians participate in regular clinical audit and reviews of clinical services.

C6
Health care organisations cooperate with each other and social care organisations to ensure that patients' individual needs are properly managed and met.

Developmental Standard
D2
Patients receive effective treatment and care that
a) conform to nationally agreed best practice, particularly as defined in National Service Frameworks, NICE guidance, national plans and agreed national guidance on service delivery;
b) take into account their individual requirements and meet their physical, cultural, spiritual and psychological needs and preferences;
c) are well coordinated to provide a seamless service across all organisations that need to be involved, especially social care organisations; and
d) is delivered by health care professionals who make clinical decisions based on evidence-based practice.

Third Domain – Governance
Domain Outcome
Managerial and clinical leadership and accountability, as well as the organisation's culture, systems and working practices, ensure that probity, quality assurance, quality improvement and patient safety are central components of all the activities of the health care organisation.

Core Standards
C7
Health care organisations
a) apply the principles of sound clinical and corporate governance;

b) actively support all employees to promote openness, honesty, probity, accountability, and the economic, efficient and effective use of resources;

c) undertake systematic risk assessment and risk management (including compliance with the controls assurance standards);

d) ensure financial management achieves economy, effectiveness, efficiency, probity and accountability in the use of resources;

e) challenge discrimination, promote equality and respect human rights; and

f) meet existing performance requirements.

C8

Health care organisations support their staff through

a) having access to processes which permit them to raise, in confidence and without prejudicing their position, concerns over any aspect of service delivery, treatment or management that they consider to have a detrimental effect on patient care or on the delivery of services; and

b) organisational and personal development programmes which recognise the contribution and value of staff, and address, where appropriate, under-representation of minority groups.

C9

Health care organisations have a systematic and planned approach to the management of records to ensure that, from the moment a record is created until its ultimate disposal, the organisation maintains information so that it serves the purpose it was collected for and disposes of the information appropriately when no longer required.

C10

Health care organisations

a) undertake all appropriate employment checks and ensure that all employed or contracted professionally qualified staff are registered with the appropriate bodies; and

b) require that all employed professionals abide by relevant published codes of professional practice.

C11

Health care organisations ensure that staff concerned with all aspects of the provision of health care

a) are appropriately recruited, trained and qualified for the work they undertake;

b) participate in mandatory training programmes; and

c) participate in further professional and occupational development commensurate with their work throughout their working lives.

C12
Health care organisations which either lead or participate in research have systems in place to ensure that the principles and requirements of the research governance framework are consistently applied.

Developmental Standards
D3
Integrated governance arrangements representing best practice are in place in all health care organisations and across all health communities and clinical networks.

D4
Health care organisations work together to
a) ensure that the principles of clinical governance are underpinning the work of every clinical team and every clinical service;
b) implement a cycle of continuous quality improvement; and
c) ensure effective clinical and managerial leadership and accountability.

D5
Health care organisations work together and with social care organisations to meet the changing health needs of their population by
a) having an appropriately constituted workforce with appropriate skill mix across the community; and
b) ensuring the continuous improvement of services through better ways of working.

D6
Health care organisations use effective and integrated information technology and information systems which support and enhance the quality and safety of patient care, choice and service planning.

D7
Health care organisations work to enhance patient care by adopting best practice in human resources management and continuously improving staff satisfaction.

Fourth Domain – Patient Focus

Domain Outcome
Health care is provided in partnership with patients, their carers and relatives, respecting their diverse needs, preferences and choices, and in part-

nership with other organisations (especially social care organisations) whose services impact on patient wellbeing.

Core Standards
C13

Health care organisations have systems in place to ensure that
a) staff treat patients, their relatives and carers with dignity and respect;
b) appropriate consent is obtained when required for all contacts with patients and for the use of any patient confidential information; and
c) staff treat patient information confidentially, except where authorised by legislation to the contrary.

C14

Health care organisations have systems in place to ensure that patients, their relatives and carers
a) have suitable and accessible information about, and clear access to, procedures to register formal complaints and feedback on the quality of services;
b) are not discriminated against when complaints are made; and
c) are assured that organisations act appropriately on any concerns and, where appropriate, make changes to ensure improvements in service delivery.

C15

Does not apply to dentistry.

C16

Health care organisations make information available to patients and the public on their services, provide patients with suitable and accessible information on the care and treatment they receive and, where appropriate, inform patients on what to expect during treatment, care and after-care.

Developmental Standards
D8

Health care organisations continuously improve the patient experience, based on the feedback of patients, carers and relatives.

D9

Patients, service users and, where appropriate, carers receive timely and suitable information, when they need and want it, on treatment, care, services, prevention and health promotion and are
a) encouraged to express their preferences; and

b) supported to make choices and shared decisions about their own health care.

D10

Patients and service users, particularly those with long-term conditions, are helped to contribute to planning of their care and are provided with opportunities and resources to develop competence in self-care.

Fifth Domain – Accessible and Responsive Care

Domain Outcome

Patients receive services as promptly as possible, have choice in access to services and treatments, and do not experience unnecessary delay at any stage of service delivery or of the care pathway.

Core Standards

C17

The views of patients, their carers and others are sought and taken into account in designing, planning, delivering and improving health care services.

C18

Health care organisations enable all members of the population to access services equally and offer choice in access to services and treatment equitably.

C19

Health care organisations ensure that patients with emergency health needs are able to access care promptly and within nationally agreed timescales, and all patients are able to access services within national expectations on access to services.

Developmental Standard

D11

Health care organisations plan and deliver health care which
a) reflects the views and health needs of the population served and which is based on nationally agreed evidence or best practice;
b) maximises patient choice;
c) ensures access (including equality of access) to services through a range of providers and routes of access; and
d) uses locally agreed guidance, guidelines or protocols for admission, referral and discharge that accord with the latest national expectations on access to services.

Sixth Domain – Care Environment and Amenities

Domain Outcome
Care is provided in environments that promote patient and staff wellbeing and respect for patients' needs and preferences in that they are designed for the effective and safe delivery of treatment, care or a specific function, provide as much privacy as possible, are well maintained and are cleaned to optimise health outcomes for patients.

Core Standards
C20
Health care services are provided in environments which promote effective care and optimise health outcomes by being
a) a safe and secure environment which protects patients, staff, visitors and their property, and the physical assets of the organisation; and
b) supportive of patient privacy and confidentiality.

C21
Health care services are provided in environments which promote effective care and optimise health outcomes by being well designed and well maintained with cleanliness levels in clinical and non-clinical areas that meet the national specification for clean NHS premises.

Developmental Standard
D12
Health care is provided in well designed environments that
a) promote patient and staff wellbeing, and meet patients' needs and preferences, and staff concerns; and
b) are appropriate for the effective and safe delivery of treatment, care or a specific function, including the effective control of health care associated infections.

Seventh Domain – Public Health

Domain Outcome
Programmes and services are designed and delivered in collaboration with all relevant organisations and communities to promote, protect and improve the health of the population served and reduce health inequalities between different population groups and areas.

Core Standards

C22
Health care organisations promote, protect and demonstrably improve the health of the community served, and narrow health inequalities by
a) cooperating with each other and with Local Authorities and other organisations;
b) ensuring that the local Director of Public Health's Annual Report informs their policies and practices; and
c) making an appropriate and effective contribution to local partnership arrangements including Local Strategic Partnerships and Crime and Disorder Reduction Partnerships.

C23
Health care organisations have systematic and managed disease prevention and health promotion programmes which meet the requirements of the National Service Frameworks and national plans with particular regard to reducing obesity through action on nutrition and exercise, smoking, substance misuse and sexually transmitted infections.

C24
Health care organisations protect the public by having a planned, prepared and, where possible, practised response to incidents and emergency situations which could affect the provision of normal services.

Developmental Standard

D13
Health care organisations
a) identify and act upon significant public health problems and health inequality issues, with Primary Care Trusts taking the leading role;
b) implement effective programmes to improve health and reduce health inequalities;
c) protect their populations from identified current and new hazards to health; and
d) take fully into account current and emerging policies and knowledge on public health issues in the development of their public health programmes, health promotion and prevention services for the public, and the commissioning and provision of services.

The Themes of Clinical Governance

In an effort to help dentists comply with the requirements, the Department of Health, in association with the NHS Modernisation Agency's National Primary and Care Trust Development Programme (NatPaCT), has developed a themed approach to meeting the clinical governance requirements for general dental practice. Many of the requirements will be in place already as part of the practice management framework, but may not have been perceived as relating to clinical governance. In the first chapter of *Clinical Governance in General Dental Practice*, the authors noted that: *"Clinical governance in primary dental care is nourished by the tenets of successful business practice. It draws on practice management principles, but applies additional tools…"*

The core and developmental standards have been grouped in a way that makes it easier for dentists to comply. They reflect the structures and processes found in dental practices; this cross-mapping of the HC standards has contextualised clinical governance for dentists. The themes and the requirements within each theme are summarised in Table 7-4 (pages 115 to 117).

Additional Resources

An interactive CD ROM developed by Smile-on Ltd. in association with the Kent, Surrey and Sussex Deanery in England helps dentists to comply with the seven domain framework. A unique programme for the dental team, it has been adopted by many PCTs and is in use in over 500 practices. It serves as a training tool within the practice helping all members of the team to grasp the meaning of clinical governance. The principles of quality improvement and use of the PDCA cycle discussed in Chapter 5 have been used to achieve the required standards in an inter-active format which allows all team members to be involved (Figs 7-3, 7-4, page 118).

The screen image at the stage of initial assessment and the completion feedback is presented in an easy-to-read dial display (Fig 7-5, page 119).

Table 7-4 The themes of clinical governance. Reference: Primary Care Contracting www.pcc.nhs.uk

Theme	Requirements – key actions and policies
1. Infection Control C1, C4, C10, C20, C21, D1, D12, D13	Procedures in accordance with BDA/DH Advice sheet A12 (Infection Control in Dentistry) including: • Infection control policy • Innoculation injury policy and recording of Hepatitis B immunisation status of exposure prone staff • Staff induction programme to include infection control procedures and staff training • Audit of policy compliance
2. Child Protection C2, C6, C10	• Identification and CRB checks for all staff • Child protection policy which is consistent with local and wider policies including any staff training requirements
3. Dental Radiography C1, C11, C24	Procedures and policies in accordance with the IRR (1999) and IR(ME)R (2000) including: • A quality assurance system • X-ray malfunction plan, including how to manage an unintended over-exposure • Records of staff training and updates • X-ray equipment maintenance records
4. Staff, Patient, Public and Environmental Safety C1, C4, C5, C20, C21, D12	• Significant events analysis procedures and changes to procedures initiated as a result • Compliance with Reporting of Injuries, Diseases and Dangerous Occurrences Regulations (RIDDOR) 1995 • Procedures to ensure all relevant safety alert bulletins are disseminated to staff and acted on • All medical devices are CE compliant, staff training for usage provided and incident reporting carried out • Medicines are appropriately sourced, purchased and stored including a medical emergencies drug kit • Compliance with Carriage of Dangerous Goods and Use of Transferable Pressure Equipment (Amendment) Regulations, 2005 • Hazardous Waste Regulations 2005 and the management of waste amalgam/mercury • Health and Safety at Work Act 1974 • Management of Health and Safety at Work Regulations 1999 • Workplace (Health, Safety and Welfare) Regulations 1992 • Control of Substances Hazardous to Health Regulations 2002 (Also see **Infection Control**, **Child Protection** and **Dental Radiography**)

Theme	Requirements – key actions and policies
5. Evidence-based Practice and Research C1, C3, C5, C12, D2, D11	• Relevant NICE Guidelines are followed • Clinical care is informed by other evidence-based guidelines • Existing care pathways and referral protocols are followed • Where appropriate, principles of research governance are applied
6. Prevention and Public Health C22, C23, D13	An evidence-based prevention policy for all oral diseases and conditions appropriate to the needs of the local population and consistent with local and national priorities. This should include: • Links to any existing community-based strategies • Tobacco use cessation • Alcohol consumption advice • (Also see **Infection Control, Patient, Public and Environmental Safety**)
7. Clinical Records, Patient Privacy and Confidentiality C9, C13, C20	• Staff awareness of and compliance with Data Protection Act 1998 • Caldicott Guidelines 1997, Access to Health Records 1998 and Confidentiality Code of Practice 1998 are followed • Confidentiality policy. Satisfactory arrangements for confidential discussions with patients • Data protection policy
8. Staff Involvement and Development (for all staff) C5, C7, C8, C10, C11, C21, C24, D7, D12	• Employment policies – appropriate job descriptions for all posts • Appraisal, personal development plans and links to mentoring schemes • Appropriate staff training undertaken and records of staff training maintained (e.g. customer training, equal opportunities, dealing with complaints and patient feedback) • Records of practice meetings and evidence of staff involvement • Protected time for staff meetings and clinical governance • Confidential process for staff to raise concerns about performance • Links to a local Practitioner Advice and Support Scheme (PASS) or similar • Evidence of regular basic life support training • Evidence that staff opinion is sought about practice matters (e.g. staff surveys, practice meeting)

Theme	Requirements – key actions and policies
9. Clinical Staff Requirements and Development C4, C5, C10, C11	(Items listed under **Staff Involvement and Development** also apply) All GDC requirements are met including: • GDC registration/enrolment where appropriate • Supervision of clinical staff • Continuing Professional Development requirements • Handling of complaints • Dealing with poor performance (including "whistle blowing" policy)
10. Patient Information and Involvement C3, C7, C13, C14, C16, C17, C18, C19, C21, D2, D3, D5, D8, D9, D10, D11	• Patients' and carers' views on services are sought and acted upon • Patients have opportunities to ask questions and provided with sufficient information to make informed decisions about their care • Patient information leaflets are available in languages appropriate to the local population • Well-publicised complaints system that is supportive of patients • Other patient feedback methods are available (e.g. suggestion boxes) • Evidence that practice have acted on findings of patient feedback • Information for patients on how to access NHS care in and out of hours
11. Fair and Accessible Care C7, C13, C18, C19, C21, D11	(Items listed under **Patient Information and Involvement** may also apply). • Compliance with the Race Relations (Amendment) Act 2000 and Human Rights Act 1998 • Access to interpreting services • All reasonable efforts made to comply with the Disability Discrimination Act 1995 • Emergency/urgent appointments available during the day
12. Clinical Audit and Peer Review C5, D1, D3, D4, D5	• All staff involved in identifying priorities for and involved in clinical audit or peer review • Evidence of compliance with any locally agreed requirements for clinical audit or peer review • Evidence that changes have been made where necessary, as a result of clinical audit or peer review

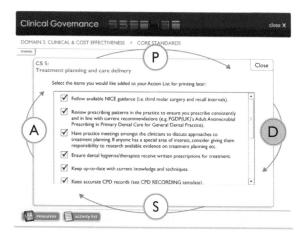

Fig 7-3 The PDSA cycle in use. This shows the "DO" stage of the cycle.

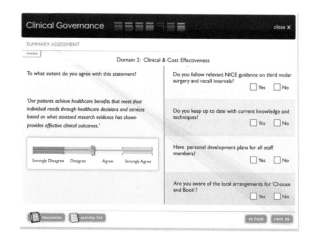

Fig 7-4 Summary data.

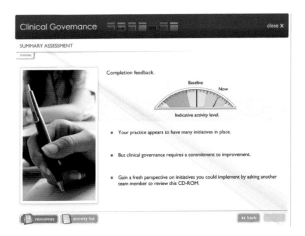

Fig 7-5 Summary data presented in a dynamic and visual format.

References

Department of Health. The new NHS: modern, dependable. London: Stationery Office, 1997.

Healthcare Commission. Standards for Better Health. Dept of Health, 2004, updated 2006.

Lilley R. Making Sense of Clinical Governance. Oxford: Radcliffe Medical Press, 1999.

National Patient Safety Agency. Medical Error. NPSA, Sept 2005.

Further Reading

D'Cruz L, Rattan R, Watson M. Understanding NHS Dentistry. New Contract Help Books, 2006.

Rattan R, Chambers R, Wakely G. Clinical Governance in General Dental Practice. Oxford: Radcliffe Publishing, 2001.

Chapter 8
Evidence-based Dentistry

Aims

The aims of this chapter are to highlight the importance and methodology of evidence-based practice and how this impacts on clinical decision making.

Outcome

As a result of reading this chapter, the reader should have an understanding of the principles of evidence-based practice and their relevance to the quality agenda.

Introduction

To ensure that we provide a quality clinical service to our patients, we should be asking four questions:
1. Are we doing things in the right way?
2. What is the evidence relating to our prescribing preferences?
3. Is the clinical care and treatment that we are providing effective?
4. How can we ensure that necessary changes are put into clinical practice?

Writing in the Journal of the American Dental Association (ADA) in 2004, Ismail and Bader advised that: "In developing appropriate treatment plans, dentists should combine the patient's treatment needs and preferences with the best available scientific evidence, in conjunction with the dentist's clinical expertise. To keep pace with other health professions in building a strong evidence-based foundation, dentistry will require significant investments in clinical research and education to evaluate the best currently available evidence in dentistry and to identify new information needed to help dentists provide optimal care to patients."

To achieve quality in the advice we give patients, we rely on the currency and the validity of our knowledge and understanding of clinical dentistry and the value judgements of the patient (Fig 8-1). The principles and methods of evidence-based dentistry (EBD) give us the opportunity to apply relevant research findings for the benefit of our patients.

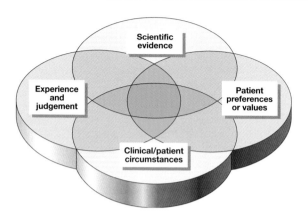

Fig 8-1 Evidence-based decision making process.
Source: Journal of contemporary dental practice 2002;vol.3:no.3.

To answer the questions posed at the beginning of this chapter would require the reader to be familiar with the thousands of articles and references published each year and to systematically collate, interpret and apply the information contained in them. It is said that many clinical decisions are opinions based on personal values and available resources – but there is now a shift towards the evidence-based approach (Fig 8-2).

In his speech at the ADA's symposium on EBD, president Eugene Sekiguchi remarked that: "Given the dramatic increase in the amount of information available about oral health, and the probability that much of this information is unsubstantiated, the need for an evidence-based approach to oral healthcare and dental practice becomes greater than ever."

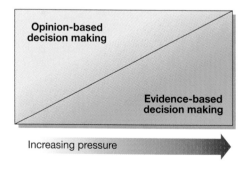

Fig 8-2 The shift from opinion-based decision making to evidence-based decision making.

The Agency for Healthcare Research and Quality (AHRQ) in the US sponsors and conducts research that provides evidence-based information on healthcare outcomes including quality, cost, usage, and access. One study looked at the use of crowns and their alternatives and noted widespread variation in prescription and cost.

The researchers concluded that if a substantial portion of the variation stems from the idiosyncratic use of crowns by dentists, the profession has a clear indication of the need to improve knowledge of treatment outcomes among practitioners.

Since there appears to be substantial disagreement about the relative life expectancies of crowns vs. their alternatives, the researchers concluded that more outcomes effectiveness research is needed, given the wide difference in the costs of alternative treatments.

Hayden, in The Journal of Dental Education (1997) goes further, and points out that the dental profession lacks basic evidence that many of the dental treatments provided are even effective. He also suggests that soon payers and patients will no longer accept anecdotal stories about quality; they will want measurement and quantification instead.

Commenting on patients' awareness of clinical issues from the Internet, Jeyanthi John, writing in the journal Evidence-based Dentistry (2003) remarked that: "It was important for all members of the dental team to be able to advise their patients about the most appropriate options and be able to back up their advice with the available evidence."

Definition

The American Dental Association defines EBD as: "An approach to oral healthcare that requires the judicious integration of systematic assessments of clinically relevant scientific evidence, relating to the patient's oral and medical condition and history, with the dentist's clinical expertise and the patient's treatment needs and preferences."

This definition, in contrast to some others, acknowledges the importance of an individual dentist's judgement in assessing the options for the patient as well as involving them in the final decision.

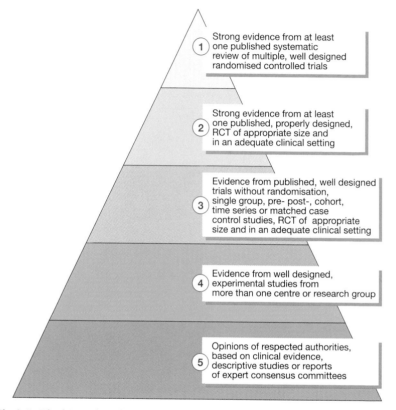

Fig 8-3 The hierarchy of evidence.

Hierarchy of Evidence

As practising clinicians we need to identify a clinical question and look for the evidence, decide if the results are believable, and how the findings can be applied to our patients. We should do this in a critical way. Rules of evidence have been established to grade evidence according to its strength.

The levels of evidence based on the classification developed by the Centre for Evidence-based Medicine is shown in Fig 8-3. Systematic reviews and randomised controlled trials (RCTs) represent the highest levels of evidence, whereas case reports and expert opinion are the lowest. Using the categories of evidence only helps classify studies based on the type of research design. The quality of each individual study still needs to be assessed for strengths and weaknesses using the techniques of critical appraisal. One way to do this is for the reader to ask some key questions (Table 8-1).

Research Design

Writing in the Journal of the Canadian Dental Association (2001), Susan Sutherland observed that: "The critical appraisal of the evidence is made easier if one understands the basic concepts of clinical research design."

Clinical research can be divided into two broad areas:
- Experimental – where the intervention is under the control of the researcher, whereas in observational studies, the researcher observes patients at a point in time (cross-sectional studies) or over time (longitudinal studies).
- Observational – where the observations are made by looking forward and gathering new data, the study is prospective; if the data already exist (for instance, in dental records or as census data), the studies are retrospective.

Table 8-1 **Questions for assessing the quality of the study**
Source: Greenhalgh, T. Assessing the methodological quality of published papers. British Medical Journal 1997;315:305-308.

Question 1: Was the study original?

Question 2: Who is the study about?
How were they recruited?
Who was included?
Who was excluded?

Question 3: Was the design sensible?
What was the intervention and what was it compared with?
What outcome was measured and how?

Question 4: Was systematic bias avoided or minimised?

Question 5: Was the assessment blind?

Question 6: Were preliminary statistical questions dealt with?
Sample size?
Duration of follow up?
Completeness of follow up?

Experimental Studies

Experimental studies can be either controlled (there is a comparison group) or uncontrolled. Uncontrolled studies provide very weak evidence; they should not be used to guide practice. They may be carried out early in an area of research to explore the safety of a new intervention, to identify unanticipated effects and to gather baseline data for the planning of more definitive trials.

Observational Studies

RCTs cannot answer all clinical questions. There are situations where they may not be necessary, appropriate, ethical or feasible. In general, questions of therapy are best answered by RCTs, whereas questions of diagnosis, prognosis and causation may be best addressed by observational studies. Also known as epidemiological studies, they are frequently undertaken in dentistry, and can be challenging to design and execute, in terms of controlling bias. It is very important to use critical appraisal methods to assess validity when assessing the evidence from observational studies.

Randomised Controlled Trials (RCTs)

RCTs are the gold standard by which all clinical research is judged because RCTs minimise bias. In any study involving people there are potentially many unknown factors, genetic or lifestyle factors that can have a bearing on the outcome. Randomisation reduces the risk that these unknown factors will be *seriously* unbalanced in the various study groups. It is randomisation that makes the RCT one of the most powerful tools of scientific research.

Another other key feature of RCTs is blinding. The "double-blind" trial is one in which both the researcher and the patient do not know whether the patient is in the experimental group or in the control group.

Published studies indicate that 37% of medical interventions are supported by evidence from an RCT and 76% were supported by compelling evidence.

Basing important clinical decisions on single trials can be risky. Because of the numbers of patients needed to detect small to moderate differences for clinically important outcome measures, definitive answers may not be found in single studies, unless they are well-designed large sample trials, which are rarely carried out in dentistry. When the information from all relevant trials addressing the same question is combined using well-established, rigorous methodology, the result is a *systematic review*. Systematic reviews are considered the highest level in the evidence hierarchy at the apex of the pyramid.

126

For example, in 2003, the American Academy of Periodontology formulated clinically relevant, focused questions and developed a protocol for systematic reviews. Reviewers systematically searched online databases and print journals and contacted authors, journal editors and industry experts. For each included study, the reviewers determined the level of evidence and summarised the findings; centralised management of biostatistics provided consistency. The reviews formed the basis for development of consensus reports that included implications for both practice and research.

Case Reports
Case studies are relegated to the base of the evidence pyramid. Case reports are often used to describe a condition. The observations reflected in them are collected in an uncontrolled, unsystematic manner. Although the findings cannot be generalised to a larger population of patients, they do nevertheless form the basis of inter-professional discussions, the wider context of which may yield information supported by higher level evidence. The description of specific cases may prompt further inquiry and then allow hypotheses to be developed leading to more robustly designed studies.

Sources of Evidence

Evidence is available from a wide range of sources.

Colleagues
Iqbal and Glenny's survey (2002) involving 300 general dental practitioners in the north-west of England showed that 60% of the respondents turned to friends and colleagues in the profession for help and advice when faced with clinical uncertainties. The limitation of this source is that a colleague's opinion is just that, and is at the lowest level of the hierarchy unless supported by other higher levels of evidence. Experts and specialists also provide a useful source, but not all may agree on treatment options.

Journals and Books
It is estimated that there are over 900 dental journals available worldwide. The busy practitioner must select and read the most relevant publications in order to keep abreast of current developments. The summary pages found in many journals provide a quick reference guide as do supplements which focus on a particular aspect of clinical practice.

Professional journals have a clear advantage over books in that the information presented is usually more up to date although long lead times can compromise the validity of some articles and papers. Many journals can also be read on the Internet and will provide e-mail alerts to subscribers so that papers may be reviewed and read online.

The Internet
There is an enormous amount of information available on the worldwide web. With so many references and citations, it is not easy for anyone to source information quickly unless you access a known site. There is also a great deal of spoof information on the Internet, and this can be misleading. Clinicians may be able to recognise the more spurious claims made for certain treatments, but patients cannot.

Electronic Databases
The specialist databases include Medline which indexes a wide range of journals. It is widely recognised as the premier source of medical literature. It contains over 11 million references and about 80% of these are English Language abstracts. A staggering 400,000 references are added each year! The search facility allows users to search for articles using key words and phrases and a search help facility is available on site for new users.

In his editorial in 2005 entitled EBD – Everybody's Dentistry, Derek Richards, editor of Evidence-based Dentistry noted that: "Although Medline shows a four-fold increase in the numbers of randomised trials from 1100 per year in 1975 to 5087 in 2004, both the size and quality of these continue to disappoint…" He stresses the importance of a quantitative and qualitative approach to evidence-based practice.

Dedicated Organisations
Organisations dedicated to producing high-quality evidence to support clinical decision making include the Cochrane Collaboration which is an international network that maintains an electronic database of systematic reviews and RCTs, and the National Library for Health (NeLH) which provides a digital library for healthcare professionals.

These organisations use stringent criteria to review evidence from research and provide a "bottom line" on the subject. As Jeyanthi John observed in her article "Sources of Evidence" published in Evidence-based Dentistry: "Sometimes the bottom line is that there is no bottom line." Support for this observation is easily found; a recent article by Tavender (2005) in Evidence-based Dentistry looked at the evidence for six-monthly recalls for patients and concluded that: "There is insufficient evidence to support or refute the practice of encouraging patients to attend for dental check-ups at 6-monthly intervals."

The Centre for Reviews and Dissemination (CRD) was established in January 1994, and aims to provide research-based information about the effects of interventions used in health and social care. It has three databases, but the one relevant to dentistry is the Database of Abstracts of Reviews of Effectiveness (DARE). It contains summaries of systematic reviews which have met strict quality criteria and includes reviews about the effects of interventions. DARE is one of the databases included in the Cochrane Library, so if you have searched the Cochrane Library, records from DARE will automatically be included in your search results.

One example related to dentistry is the April 1999 publication Effective Healthcare (Vol.5, issue 2), which was devoted to dental restorations and offered guidance on the use of different restorative materials. The 12-page report is an excellent summary of the range of restorative materials and techniques and their clinical effectiveness. It is available in PDF from the CRD website: http://www.york.ac.uk/inst/crd/index.htm.

Clinical Guidelines

The Institute of Medicine in the US defines clinical guidelines as: "Systematically developed statements to assist practitioners and patients in arriving at appropriate healthcare for specific clinical circumstances." They bridge the gap between theory and practice, but the evidence suggests that only about 50% of dentists support the development and implementation of clinical guidelines – the barrier appears to be the belief that guidelines reduce professional autonomy.

Examples of guidelines available include the range of publications by the Faculty of General Dental Practitioners (FGDP) in London, which includes guidelines on clinical record keeping, radiography, and the prescribing of antibiotics. The role of NICE in the UK in this context is discussed in Chapter 7.

The Canadian Collaboration on Clinical Practice Guidelines in Dentistry is the national, autonomous organisation responsible for the development of guidelines for Canadian dentists. The recommendations are graded A–C:
Grade A – this recommendation requires evidence from at least one randomised controlled trial as part of a body of literature of overall good quality and consistency addressing the specific recommendation.

Grade B – this requires evidence from well conducted clinical studies when there are no randomised clinical trials on the topic of recommendation, or, small randomised trials with uncertain results (and moderate to high risk of error). *Grade C* – recommends evidence obtained from expert committee reports, or opinions and/or clinical experiences of respected authorities.

The Scottish Intercollegiate Guidelines Network (SIGN) was formed in 1993 with the objective of improving the quality of healthcare for patients in Scotland by reducing variation in practice and outcome, through the development and dissemination of national clinical guidelines containing recommendations for effective practice based on current evidence. The membership of SIGN includes dentistry. Since January 2005 SIGN has been part of NHS Quality Improvement Scotland. At the time of writing, guidelines are available on the management of impacted third molars and caries prevention in high-risk children. Unlike the Canadian grading system, SIGN uses four grades of recommendation ranging from A–D which reflect the evidence level available to support the publication of the guidelines. Grade A would be attached to evidence that resulted from a systematic review.

In 1999, the Canadian Dental Association helped found the Canadian Collaboration on Clinical Practice Guidelines, which is now considered to be one of the world's leading organisations in this respect.

Having guidelines is one thing, but their acceptance into everyday practice is another. In 2003, a paper was published bearing the title: "Does the dental profession know how to care for the primary dentition?" It referred to the guidelines issued by the British Society of Paediatric Dentistry (BSPD) on the restoration of carious primary molars. The authors, Milsom et al, found that a large number of experienced practitioners had created their own sets of guidelines independently of each other, believing it better to leave the untreated carious tooth to exfoliate rather than treat with a stainless steel crown.

A commentary on this paper observed that "these guidelines were no doubt developed in good faith" by the members of the BSPD, but that "a large number of practitioners felt the BSPD guidelines did not fit with the context of their practice." It was acknowledged that: "There was no scientific research to back this decision, only clinical intuition based on years of continuing care experience of hundreds, if not thousands of children."

Andrew Toy is an experienced dental practitioner with a keen interest in clinical education. He cites Donald Schön, author of *The Reflective Practitioner*, whose view is that professionals are "inherently artistic" in their decision-making. They combine facts with experience and apply them to the care of an individual patient. Toy suggests that "In general dental practice, the decisions we make every minute of our working day are usually intuitive, a mixture of both the science and the art of dentistry." It is a view many of us in practice would endorse.

PICO

PICO is an acronym for patient problem, intervention, comparison and outcome. The PICO model is a framework that facilitates decision-making in everyday practice. The use of the framework is best illustrated by a clinical example: consider a male adult 25-year-old patient, who is concerned about discolouration on his upper anterior teeth which have all been root treated some years ago as a result of a traumatic injury during his teens. He reports that he is getting married in two weeks and requests a dentist's opinion and advice about what he is able to do to improve the appearance of his teeth before the wedding.

The process of formulating the question begins with the definition of the problem, consideration of the intervention, a comparative assessment of another option and the clinical outcome (Fig 8-4).

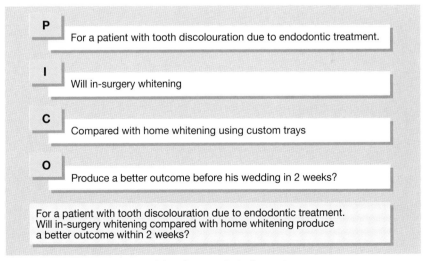

P For a patient with tooth discolouration due to endodontic treatment.

I Will in-surgery whitening

C Compared with home whitening using custom trays

O Produce a better outcome before his wedding in 2 weeks?

For a patient with tooth discolouration due to endodontic treatment. Will in-surgery whitening compared with home whitening produce a better outcome within 2 weeks?

Fig 8-4 Using the PICO model to frame a clinical question.

Another example would be a patient who is concerned about the toxicity of amalgam having sourced some information on the subject from the Internet. The patient asks the dentist for advice on what should be done, but does not want the restorations replaced unless there is good reason to do so. This is a different scenario to the one described above because the choice is between intervention and no intervention, but the PICO framework can still be used here.

The question to ask in this example would be: "For the patient with existing amalgam restoration (problem), will leaving the restorations *in situ* (intervention), compared with replacing her amalgams (comparison) result in no adverse effects to her general health?"

Clinical Decision Making

Clinical decision making is a complex process which involves diagnosis and assessment, the formulation and discussion of treatment options, dentist and patient values and related factors such as time and cost culminating in the delivery of a negotiated treatment with the informed consent of the patient. The process is summed up in Fig 8-5.

In clinical practice, we interpret how a guideline should be applied in a particular clinical situation. The condition covered by the guideline may differ in some way from the one presenting, but we must also respect that the patient's perception and values are important. A guideline may suggest a certain treatment, but the patient may have other preferences and may attach a different value to the outcome and/or other consequences of the treatment than those indicated in the guideline.

Variation

Substantial variation in dentists' treatment decisions and treatments provided has been identified in many studies and is recognised amongst clinicians. This variation has been documented at all levels in clinical practice. It has been identified at the practice level by looking at dentists' practice patterns, at the level of treatment planning for individual patients, and also at the level of the individual tooth. This variation may result from:
- ambiguity of clinical data
- variations in its interpretation
- uncertainty about relations between clinical information and presence of disease
- uncertainty about effects of treatment.

The effect of this uncertainty has been described by Kay and Nuttall (1995) as perceptual and judgemental variation. The former occurs when treatment decisions differ as a result of perception of the condition and the latter when dentists' opinions about appropriate treatment differ, but their perception of the condition is similar. They argue that when positively viewed, treatment variation between dentists is the result of a mature decision-making process affected by differing factors in each treatment case.

Factors that contribute to the variation in clinical decision-making include:

1. Skill and diligence in conducting the examination
2. Diagnostic criteria employed
3. Beliefs about course of the disease
4. Beliefs about risk factors for disease
5. Beliefs about treatment effectiveness
6. Style of patient interaction.

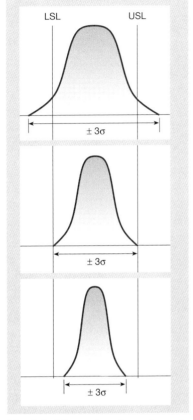

Fig 8-5 Narrowing the variance in clinical decision making.
(LSL = Lower specification limit, USL = Upper specification limit)

Decision analysis, continuous quality improvement, and practice guidelines are all aimed at narrowing this variance (Fig 8-5), and shifting upwards the bell-shaped curve of treatment distribution.

Theory of Innovation

In 1995, the fourth edition of Everett Rogers' book called *Diffusion of Innovations* was published. In it he describes his "adoption curve" which is based on his earlier work in the 1960s. According to Rogers, time and spread

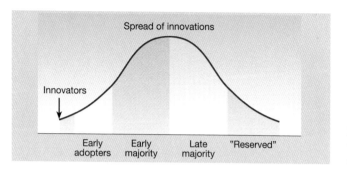

Fig 8-6 Rogers' theory of spread of innovation.

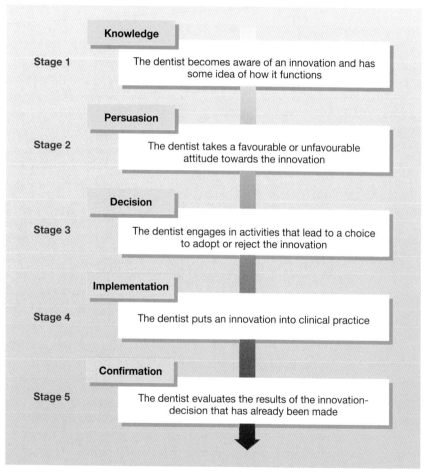

Fig 8-7 Accepting innovation in practice.

follows a pattern – the laggards or "reserved" at the end of a diffusion process that identifies innovators, early adopters, and early and late majorities in the professional community (Fig 8-6). The five stages of innovation acceptance in practice are shown in Fig 8-7.

The theory illustrates why the adoption of new ideas and working methods in clinical practice often takes time to filter through to everyday practice.

Stacey's Matrix

Ralph Stacey is professor of management and director of the Complexity and Management Centre, at the University of Hertfordshire. He proposed a matrix to help with decision making using two dimensions: the degree of certainty and the level of agreement (Fig 8-8).

The x-axis of this diagram shows the level of certainty/predictability – absolute certainty on the left and no predictability on the right. The y-axis represents the level of agreement with high agreement at the bottom and little agreement at the top of this axis.

Adapting this model to clinical decision making, we can describe two distinct features in relation to clinical conditions: the degree of certainty about the effect of management (evidence) and the degree of agreement among dentists about how to manage the conditions.

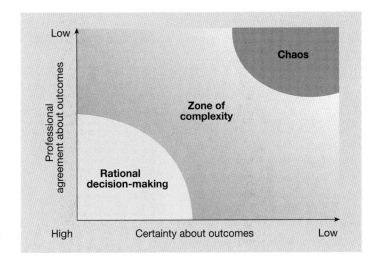

Fig 8-8
The Stacey diagram.

When faced with a condition where we are uncertain about the effect of treatment, we may not agree about its best management; this belongs to the chaotic part of the clinical spectrum and falls into the top right zone of the matrix. Between these two extremes, we attend to complex conditions.

Simple conditions have a high degree of certainty and a high degree of agreement about best management. This falls into the "rational decision-making" zone of the Stacey matrix – dentists will agree on the treatment plan and feel in control of its delivery with predictable results. Clinical decision making in this zone is easy; we are in the comfort zone of predictable outcomes. If ever challenged, we would enjoy the comfort of professional consensus. On other occasions, the picture is more complex – there is less certainty and we work under demanding conditions reviewing and re-assessing complex treatment plans. Occasionally and reluctantly, though hopefully not very often, we may transcend into the unknown where our decisions may not bear scientific scrutiny but where experience leads the decision making process and where we all have cases to support our decisions.

The prescribing tendencies amongst clinicians will vary – least in the zone where agreement and certainty are high and most at the chaotic end of the matrix. At first, it may appear that one way to reduce this variability is to encourage the development of clinical guidelines, but the further we move away from the bottom left corner of this matrix, the more complex the condition becomes and the less likely it is that we can develop an agreed clinical guideline. Nonetheless, these zones are the very zones in which we wish to reduce prescribing variations!

Summary

Clinical decision is summarised by the process depicted in Fig 8-9. It is affected by:
- the dentist-patient relationship
- the level of patient involvement
- the patient's perspective on the value of treatment
- the dentist's personal values
- the risk/benefit ratio
- the patient's financial resources.

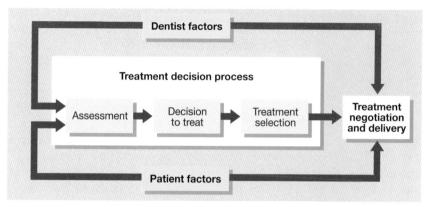

Fig 8-9 A model of the treatment decision process. Modified from Bader and Shugars, 1992.

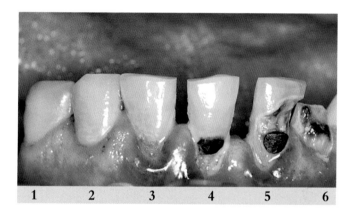

Fig 8-10 A clinical decision-making challenge.
Photograph by kind permission of Dr Douglas Bratthall, University of Malmo, Sweden.

1. A tooth surface without caries.
2. The first signs of demineralisation, a small "white spot" has been formed (initial caries, incipient caries). It is not yet a cavity, the surface is still hard. With proper measures, the caries process can be halted here and even reversed.
3. The enamel surface has broken down. There is a "lesion" with a soft floor.
4. A restoration is in place, but as can be seen, the demineralisation has not been stopped and the lesion is surrounding the amalgam restoration. It is sometimes called "Secondary caries" but in fact, it is usually the "same" disease that is in progress.
5. The demineralisation has progressed and is undermining the tooth.
6. The tooth has fractured – the consequence of a process which could have been arrested at an early stage.

Qualitative research suggests that the personality of the clinician also plays an important role in clinical behaviour. Some dentists will feel the urge to intervene and patients will receive "treatment" whilst others may prefer to take a "watch, wait and review approach". The two groups run the risk of being accused of over treating or supervised neglect. In reality, they are exercising their clinical judgement and in the absence of high level evidence which group can we say is right? The dentition shown in Fig 8-10 invites clinical intervention. What would you do to which tooth and why?

The majority of the dental research today is based on quantitative data. In *The Reflective Practitioner*, Schön comments that this research produces solutions for the problems of the *"hard, high ground"*. Therefore, it is inherently difficult to apply its results to his *"swampy lowlands"* of professional practice. To deliver quality care to our patients, we must interpret the clinical evidence and any resulting guidelines in relation to the patient and the situation.

References

Bader JD, Shugars DA. Understanding dentists' restorative treatment decisions. J Public Health Dent 1992;52:102-110.

Hayden W. Dental health services research utilizing comprehensive clinical databases and information technology. J Dent Educ 1997;61;47-55.

Iqbal A, Glenny AM. General dental practitioners' knowledge of and attitudes towards evidence based practice. Br Dent J 2002;193:587-591.

Ismail A, Bader J. Evidence-based dentistry in clinical practice. J Am Dent Assoc 2004;135:78-83.

John J. Sources of evidence. Evid Based Dent 2003;4:91-93.

Kay EJ, Nuttall NM. Clinical decision making: an art or a science? Part III. To treat or not to treat? Br Dent J 1995;178:153-155.

Milsom KM, Tickle M, King D. Does the dental profession know how to care for the primary dentition? Br Dent J 2003;195:301-303.

Richards D. Everybody's Dentistry (Editorial). Evid Based Dent 2005;6(3):57.

Rogers E. Diffusion of innovations. 4th edn. New York: Free Press, 1995.

Schön DA. The Reflective Practitioner: how professionals think in action. Arena, 1991.

Sheldon T, Treasure E. Dental Restoration: what type of filling? Effective Health Care 1999;5:2.

Sutherland SE, Matthews DC, Fendrich P. Clinical Practice Guidelines in Dentistry. J Can Dent Assoc 2001;67:448-452.

Tavender E. Insufficient evidence to support or refute the need for 6-monthly dental check-ups. Evid Based Dent 2005;6:62-63.

Chapter 9
Service Quality

Aims

This chapter aims to stress the importance of service elements in the delivery of quality care in everyday practice and to review the popular service-quality models which apply to dental practice.

Outcome

Having read this chapter, the reader should have a better understanding of what constitutes service quality.

Introduction

Organisations survive and prosper through meeting the needs of customers. High service standards contribute much to this success and, according to David Garvin of Harvard Business School it means: "Pleasing customers, not just protecting them from annoyance."

John Tschohl, described by Time magazine as the guru of customer service and now president of the Service Quality Institute, states that: "Providing exceptional customer service" should be "at the top of your list of corporate goals. While quality, price, and speed are important to customers, service is the icing on the cake. It will give you a competitive edge and keep your customers coming back to you."

Abrams et al (1986) compared dentist and patient assessments of dental restoration quality. They concluded that: "Simply practising dentistry with a high degree of technical expertise will not necessarily convince the patient that he has received high–quality dental care. Other less technical aspects of dental care are recognised as being barometers of quality of dental treatment. Practitioners should not lose sight of the human and psychological aspects of care, and keep in mind that they are integral components of quality in dental treatment." Many of these aspects relate to service quality.

There has been a stream of research into aspects of service quality and it has been conceptualised in two different ways:

1. The Nordic perspective, as articulated by Grönroos (1984), defines the dimensions of service quality as consisting of functional aspects (e.g. intangible benefits) and technical ones (e.g. the delivery of the service). These dimensions are viewed as the main properties of perceived service quality.

2. The second concept is the American one, as exemplified by the work of Parasuraman et al (1988), and revolves around the SERVQUAL model which defines service quality as the outcome of effective service delivery which occurs when customers receive service that is superior to their expectations.

According to these authors, service quality is an attitude formed by customers by comparing prior expectations of the service and their perceptions of the actual service performance. In other words, perceptions of service quality are based on the evaluation of service delivery in comparison to pre-consumption expectations, i.e. the disconfirmation model.

Details of these two approaches are presented later in this chapter.

Definition

Service quality can be defined in many ways. It is the difference between the patients' expectations for service performance prior to the encounter and their perceptions of the service actually received.

Other perspectives on service quality include:

- Service quality is superiority or excellence as perceived by the customer (Peters and Austin, 1985).
- The delivery of excellent or superior service relative to customer expectations (Zeithaml and Bitner, 1996).
- Quality is behaviour – an attitude – that says you will never settle for anything less than the best in service for your stakeholders, whether they are customers, the community, your stockholders or colleagues with whom you work every day (Harvey, 1995).
- (Quality is) providing a better service than the customer expects (Lewis, 1989).

Elements of Service Quality

Dr Michael Kendrick is a well known international consultant and the former Director of the Institute for Leadership and Community Development in the US. He has identified 30 elements of service quality (Table 9-1), which "taken together … should enhance the probability that a service actually benefits the people it was intended to serve."

Many of these elements can be applied to everyday practice and this list is a valuable checklist against which practices can evaluate their service quality.

Service Quality Models

There are a number of service quality models which can be applied to dental practice. The following examples are given:

Grönroos Model

Christian Grönroos' definition of service is: "An activity or series of activities of more or less intangible nature that normally, but not necessarily, take place in interactions between the customer and service employees and/or systems of the service provider, which are provided as solutions to customer problems."

Grönroos' model illustrates how the quality of a given service is perceived by customers by looking at two dimensions:

• *Technical quality*
This is *what* the consumer receives, the technical outcome of a process. It is the haircut if you're a barber, the advice if you're a solicitor or the ceramic onlay if you're a dentist.

• *Functional quality*
How the consumer receives the technical outcome. Grönroos calls it "expressive performance of a service". It has also been described as process quality; it is about *how* the service is delivered that is evaluated by the patient.

All members of the service team and the general atmosphere have an impact on patient satisfaction.

Grönroos suggested that, in the context of services, functional quality is generally perceived to be more important than technical quality, assuming that the service is provided at a technically satisfactory level. He also points out that the functional quality dimension can be perceived in a very subjective manner. The complete model is shown in Fig 9-1.

143

Table 9-1 **Kendrick's 30 elements of service quality** (continued over page)

Kendrick's 30 elements
1. The regard and value the agency extends to consumers.
2. The loyalty and fidelity held by service providers to those served.
3. The degree of understanding present by those served.
4. The extent to which consumers are understood in terms of their needs.
5. The extent to which the agency individualises services.
6. The level of consumer participation and guidance in regards to what is happening with and for them.
7. The relevance of service practices to people's needs and preferences.
8. The extent to which the service respects and strengthens the person's autonomy and self determination.
9. The extent to which the person is assisted in maintaining or strengthening their community.
10. The extent to which the person is supported in having and managing personal relationships.
11. The provision to consumers of just the right amount and intensity of support.
12. The extent to which the agency addresses the person's development, growth, and competencies.
13. The presence of appropriate protection and safeguards for the person's vital needs.
14. The extent to which the agency preserves and nurtures the person's natural and informal supports.
15. Respect for the rights of the person and support for the person to exercise these rights.
16. The extent to which the service and agency processes are understood and meaningful to the consumer.
17. The service should be affordable.
18. The service should adapt as individual needs change.
19. The person is not stigmatised through association with the service.
20. The service should be coordinated with other aspects of the person's life.
21. The level of appropriate acknowledgment and support for the existential, emotional and spiritual struggles of the person served.

Table 9-1 **Kendrick's 30 elements of service quality** (continued)

Kendrick's 30 elements

22. Adequate levels of structure, consistency and dependability of service.
23. When supervision is needed, it should be properly targeted, enhancing, and empowering for the person.
24. The extent to which consumers' lives are encouraged to be as normal as possible.
25. That the interests and needs of the person served are not supplanted by the interests of the caregiver or the agency.
26. Consumers should not be subjected to involuntary interruptions in their home and work life.
27. The person should have effective access to independent and competent advocacy, allies and legal advice.
28. The extent to which the agency provides compensating supports to help consumers offset practical disadvantages they may face in community living.
29. The service should be conveniently located and accessible.
30. The service should have integrity, honesty, and authenticity

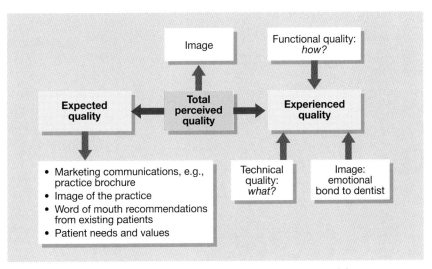

Fig 9-1 An adaptation of Grönroos' "Total perceived quality" model.

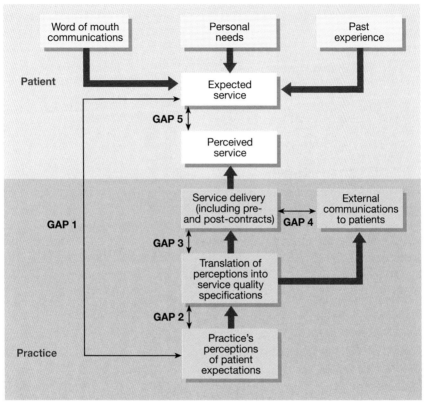

Fig 9-2 The gap model for service quality in general practice.

The Gap Model

The gap model of service quality by Parasuraman et al (1985) indicates that consumer perceptions of quality are influenced by four gaps occurring in the internal process of service delivery:

- Gap 1: Not knowing what our patients expect – the difference between patient expectations and the dentist's perceptions of these expectations.
- Gap 2: Not selecting the right service design – the difference between the dentist's perceptions of patient expectations and the service quality specifications.
- Gap 3: Not delivering to service standards – the difference between service specifications and *actual* service delivery.

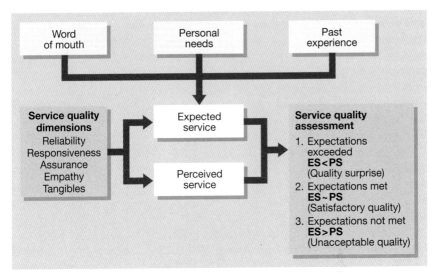

Fig 9-3 Perceived service quality.

- Gap 4: Not matching performance to promises – the difference between the service delivery and what is communicated, through practice brochures, websites and newsletters for example, about the service available to patients.

Gap 5 results from the sum of degree and direction of Gaps 1–4 and is defined as:
- Gap 5: Perceived service quality – the difference between consumer expectations and consumer perceptions.

The outcome of the practice-patient interaction depends on to what extent expectations have been met (Fig 9-3). The gaps and some reasons why they may arise are summarised in Table 9-2.

SERVQUAL Model
SERVQUAL is the tool for improving service quality. From the results of a set of about 100 questions Parasuraman et al (1985) concluded that consumers perceive service quality by comparing expectations to performance and evaluate the quality of the service in different dimensions.

The five basic dimensions are:
- Reliability: The ability to perform a promised service dependently and accurately.

Table 9-2 **Service quality gaps and possible causes**

Gap 1 Not knowing what customers expect	Lack of a marketing orientation. Inadequate upward communication (from front line contact staff to management). "Dentists know best" philosophy.
Gap 2 The wrong service quality standards	Inadequate commitment to service quality. Lack of perception of feasibility – "it cannot be done". Lack of understanding of importance. The absence of goal setting.
Gap 3 The service performance gap	Role ambiguity and role conflict – unsure of what your remit is and how it fits with others. Poor employee fit – the wrong person or system for the job. Inappropriate or lack of perceived control – too much or too little control. Lack of teamwork.
Gap 4 When promises made do not match actual delivery	When promises made to patients fail to match actual delivery – sometimes as a result of exaggerated claims.

- Responsiveness: A willingness to help customers and to provide support services.
- Assurance: The knowledge and courtesy of employees and their ability to inspire trust and confidence.
- Empathy: The caring, individual attention a firm provides its customers.
- Tangibles: The appearance of the physical facilities, up to date equipment, and appearance of the team.

Based on these quality dimensions Parasuraman et al (1988) developed a series of standard questionnaires to measure the stated gaps and to what extent they exist respectively in a given organisation. These questionnaires address the different roles like customers (Gap 5), management (Gap 1 and 2), and service contact personnel (Gap 3 and 4).

The recipients of the questionnaires were later asked to allocate 100 points among these five dimensions in order to be able to rank the importance of the respected dimension. This qualitative study identified reliability as the

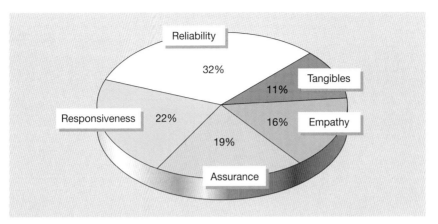

Fig 9-4 Relative importance of service dimensions when respondants allocate 100 points. Reproduced with permission from A. Parasuraman, University of Miami.

most important dimension used by customers in evaluating service quality, regardless of the service industry, with responsiveness being next. Tangibles has the lowest influence on overall service quality (Fig 9-4).

The SERVQUAL model has been adapted by other workers to cover different areas. This list and its application to dental practice is summarised in Table 9-3.

A significant extension was undertaken by Zeithaml and Bitner (1996). By expanding the SERVQUAL technique to include the relationship among customer service expectations, service level antecedents, perceived service, service quality, customer satisfaction, and other depending parameters, they extended the Gap 5 concept and called it the zone of tolerance (Fig 9-5).

In this case, the customers' expectations of service quality are measured at three levels, namely:
• Desired Service: The level of service representing a blend of what customers believe can be and should be provided.
• Adequate Service: The minimum level of service customers are willing to accept during the process of service delivery.
• Predicted Service: This is the level of service customers believe they are likely to receive.

According to Zeithaml and Bitner, customers recognise variances in service performance and the extent to which they are willing to accept this

Table 9-3 **An expanded service quality model**

Tangibles	The physical appearance of the practice, inside and outside. The cleanliness of the uniforms and the quality of practice information booklets, notepaper and other communication channels.
Reliability	The ability of the team to undertake the promised service dependably and accurately.
Responsiveness	The willingness to help patients and provide prompt service.
Competence	The possession of the required knowledge and skills to deliver the service and perform the clinical tasks.
Courtesy	The politeness, friendliness and consideration shown to patients by members of the team.
Credibility	The trustworthiness, believability and honesty of those performing the service. This is often judged by inference – qualifications and practice accreditation displays.
Feeling of security	The patient feels safe and has no reason to doubt anything in the environment. Control and management of risk is also important.
Access	The dentist is approachable and easy to contact and schedule appointments in a timely manner.
Communication	The dentist listens to the patients and treatment options are explained and negotiated in a language that the patient can understand.
Understanding the customer	Efforts are made to understand the needs of the patients and to get to know their concerns and values.

variation is called the *zone of tolerance*. It is worth noting that predicted service may be the same as adequate or desired service, but is most likely to be somewhere between the two but within this zone of tolerance. We could say that so long as we work within the confines of this zone, our patients will not particularly notice service performance. Step outside the zone, then patients will notice the difference and express it as satisfaction or dissatisfaction depending on the extent and direction of variance.

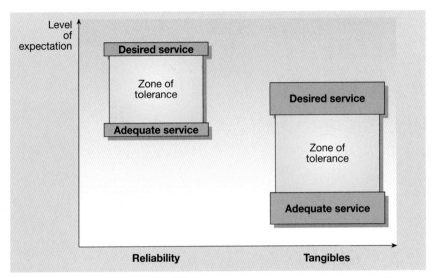

Fig 9-5 Zones of tolerance for different service dimensions. Source: Berry, LL, Parasuraman A, Zeithaml VA. Ten Lessons for Improving Service Quality. Marketing Science Institute 1993. Report no. 93-104.

Internal Service Quality

The concept of the internal marketplace is based on the notion that to have satisfied patients, the practice must also have satisfied employees. Greater employee satisfaction is more likely to result in a patient-focused practice.

Grönroos talked about "selling the firm to the employees" who are treated as "internal customers". Berry and Parasuraman use the phrase "wooing employees" to satisfy their needs through developing and motivating them.

The focus on employee satisfaction can be attributed to the fact that human acts of performance are what patients buy. Many of these were explored in the first book in this series, *The Business of Dentistry*, and the author cited the work of Heskett et al (1997) and the concept of the service-profit chain which shows linkages between internal service quality, employee satisfaction, their productivity, and external customer satisfaction (Fig 9-6).

The gap analysis can be applied in the same way to the internal situation (Fig 9-7).

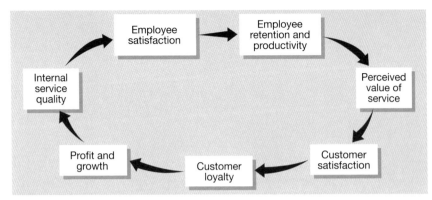

Fig 9-6 The service profit chain. Heskett, JL, Sasser, EW, Schlesinger, LA. The Service Profit Chain: How Leading Companies Link Profit and Growth to Loyalty, Satisfaction and Value. Free Press, 1997.

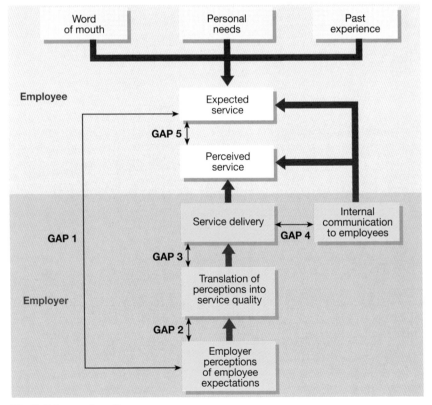

Fig 9-7 Internal quality gaps.

References

Abrams R, Ayers C, Vogt Petterson M. Quality assessment of dental restorations: a comparison by dentists and patients. Community Dent Oral Epidemiol 1986;14:317-319.

Berry L, Parasuraman A. Marketing Services: competing through quality. New York: Free Press, 1991.

Grönroos C. A service quality model and its marketing implications. Eur J Mark 1984;18(4):37-44.

Grönroos C. From marketing mix to relationship marketing: towards a paradigm shift in marketing. Management Dec 1994;32(2):4-20.

Harvey T. Service quality: the culprit and the cure. Bank Mark 1995;June:24-28.

Lewis B. Quality in the service sector: a review. Int J Bank Mark 1989;7(5):4-12.

Parasuraman A, Zeithaml V, Berry L. A conceptual model of service quality and its implications for future research. J Mark 1985;Fall:41-50.

Parasuraman A, Zeithaml V, Berry L. Servqual: a multi-item scale for measuring consumer perceptions of service quality. J Retailing 1988;64:12-37.

Peters T, Austin N. A Passion for Excellence: the leadership difference. New York: Random House, 1985.

Zeithaml V, Bitner MJ. Services Marketing. New York: McGraw-Hill, 1996.

Zeithaml V, Parasuraman A, Berry L. Delivering Quality Service: balancing customer perceptions and expectations. New York: Free Press, 1990.

Chapter 10
Business Implications

Aims

The aims of this chapter are to consider the impact of quality in the context of the business of dentistry.

Outcome

The reader should appreciate the business benefits of implementing quality improvements in general dental practice.

Introduction

General practice is a business enterprise that has identified a need and organises internal and external resources to meet that need in a clinically effective and ethically sound manner. Profitability is one indicator of how well the task has been carried out. Inherent in this is the need to understand the requirements of the patient and to have available the range of clinical products, techniques, facilities and services to meet those requirements.

These should be delivered in a consistent way, preferably exceeding patient expectations. Patient satisfaction is part of a cyclic process that is summarised in Fig 10-1.

Delivering Value

It was Walter A. Shewhart, the originator of the PDCA cycle, as discussed in Chapter 5, who noted that: "Price has no meaning without a measure of the quality being purchased."

Quality and cost are intimately related and value is the combination of the quality of a product and the cost at which that level of quality is achieved (Fig 10-2, Fig 10-3).

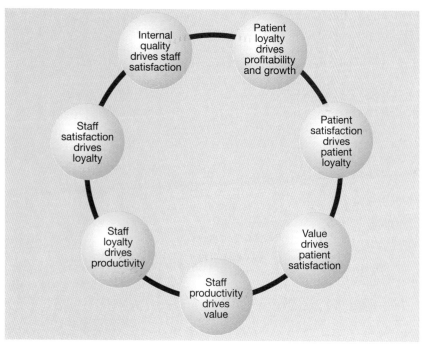

Fig 10-1 The multi-linkages of the service-profit chain.

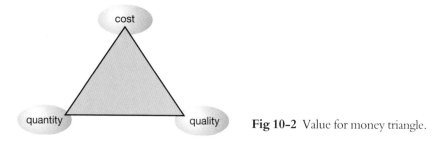

Fig 10-2 Value for money triangle.

We have established in earlier chapters that it is difficult for patients to measure the technical quality, and that patients will rely on indicators which will assist them in evaluating that quality.

In discussing the cost and quality of clinical treatments with our patients, we frequently refer to content quality. From this technical/content perspective, high value clinical care results from the most efficient expenditure of resources to achieve an established high level of clinical quality. Also, most dentists would agree that to achieve higher quality would often involve incurring additional costs – laboratory fees being just one example.

CQI theory takes a different, somewhat counter-intuitive argument that suggests that high quality can result in lower costs, within certain limits. To illustrate the principal, we need to review five areas:

1. Quality waste.
2. Productivity.
3. Maximalism versus optimalism in the face of limited resources.
4. The effect of improving the best clinical outcome that can be achieved through the application of new technology, new medications, or new techniques.
5. Lifestyle factors and the role of preventive dentistry.

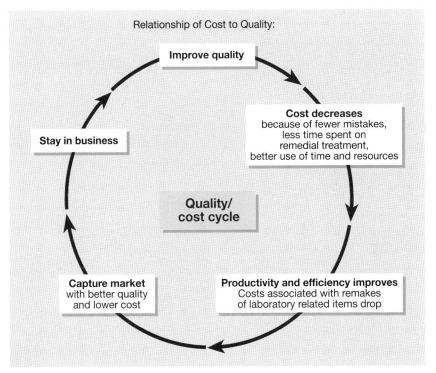

Fig 10-3 The relationship of cost to quality. Adapted from: W. Edwards Deming. Out of the Crisis: Relationship of Cost to Quality. MIT press, 1986.

Quality Waste

Low quality results when a process fails. For example, a failure in the process of recording an accurate impression of teeth prepared to receive a conventional bridge will result in an ill-fitting fixed prosthesis. The outcome brings with it a series of high costs. This bridge must now be discarded and all of the resources that went into its fabrication – in the practice and in the laboratory – are wasted. The process of impression taking may have failed for a number of reasons – Ishikawa's cause and effect diagram is a useful tool here – but one reason may be the difficulty of obtaining a homogenous mix of the impression material.

We need to ask some key questions:
1. Who pays for the discarded bridge?
2. Additional resources must be allocated to correct the deficiency. Who pays for the new work?
3. The patient may be dissatisfied with the outcome and may elect to have the treatment elsewhere. What is the cost to the reputation of the practice of a dissatisfied patient? It costs far more to attract a new patient than it costs to retain an existing one.
4. What has been the cost of the time that must be spent on dealing with the dissatisfied patient and further discussions with the laboratory?

The conclusion is self-evident – a low quality process has led directly to higher end costs. Philip Crosby describes this as *quality waste;* it represents the resources that are consumed when the output fails to meet quality expectations. The cost of poor quality is discussed in more detail later in this chapter.

Productivity

Low productivity occurs when an alternative approach will achieve the same quality using fewer resources. It differs from maximalism which achieves higher quality but at an increasingly unfavourable cost.

Optimalism and Maximalism

There are occasions in clinical practice where gains in quality may not justify the increase in practice resources both from a patient and practitioner perspective. If this is the case, clinicians will attempt to achieve an optimal level of quality for the resources consumed – which may be measured in terms of the price to the patient. In other words, they will try and maximise value, but may not achieve the ultimate quality outcome. This is optimalism and is a necessary approach when resources are finite.

From an ethical standpoint, healthcare professionals should not be placed in the position of limiting content quality on the basis of cost. Many, if not all, dentists would welcome an environment where the best possible output was achieved regardless of cost – dentists in this group are called maximalists. The undesirable result of maximalism is that the unchecked use of resources for limited benefits displaces the scope for more usefully deployed resources potentially serving more people.

It is a generalisation, but Donabedian suggests that healthcare practitioners tend to be maximalists because then they need only decide if an additional element of care will be useful. Optimal care requires the added expertise of weighing up cost and outcome of each additional element of cost – trying to evaluate the options remains one of the enduring challenges in the business of dentistry.

New Technology
Science and technology in dentistry continues to advance. New technologies provide a greater likelihood of superior clinical outcomes. The use of apex locators, ultrasound irrigation and NiTi instrumentation in endodontics are one example, and adhesive technologies another.

New technologies are assessed by Government agencies to see if they are effective and efficacious. The reference to NICE in Chapter 7 is one example of this process. New techniques are demonstrated through clinical research and reported in the medical literature before they find widespread acceptance (see Chapter 8). They change the expectations of the final output amongst practitioners and are usually associated with higher costs.

Lifestyle and Prevention
Lifestyle factors, such as diet, standard of oral hygiene and tobacco usage, have a profound impact on dental disease experience. Preventive dentistry is recognised to be significantly more cost-effective than the treatment of an established condition. Patients should be encouraged to maintain health and have access to the appropriate advice and guidance from members of the clinical team in this respect.

Quality Costs

The American Society for Quality Control defines quality costs as: "A measure of costs specifically associated with the achievement or non-achievement of product or service quality – as defined by all product or service requirements established by the company and its contracts with customers."

A more concise definition of quality costs is: "All costs incurred to help the employee do the right job every time and the cost of determining if the output is acceptable, plus any cost incurred by the organisation and the customer because the output does not meet specifications and/or customer expectations."

In general practice, direct, visible costs of poor quality include such obvious expenditures as the costs associated with inaccurate laboratory work, excessive overtime by team members (perhaps as a result of system or personal ineffectiveness as discussed in Chapter 5), clinical errors, use of outmoded technologies, faulty equipment and ineffective materials.

The indirect or latent costs of quality in general practice include the economic consequences of such intangible factors as ineffective communication amongst team members and with patients, lack of teamwork, poorly trained staff members, the financial effects of treatment errors, overdue accounts and inefficient working practices.

Return on Investment (ROI)

ROI is the ratio derived from the sum of improvement benefits divided by the sum of the costs incurred for making that improvement. For example, a 10:1 ratio means that £10.00 of benefit has resulted for every £1.00 spent.

It is difficult to measure ROI in general practice because many of the benefits that are derived as a result of quality improvement cannot be quantified in monetary terms. How can we quantify the ROI of a quality improvement initiative which prevents a complaint, damage to reputation, litigation or referral to a professional regulatory body that is empowered to suspend dentists from the register? No amount of investment would be considered too steep for preventing such an occurrence.

ROI comes from business growth and recommendations – many of which result from satisfying patient needs and exceeding their expectations. In a profession where reputation is all, the case for quality cannot always be translated into an exact ratio. Suffice it to say that any investment should return the investor a handsome multiple of the initial and ongoing investment.

The Malcolm Baldrige National Quality Award identifies companies who are committed to total quality management. In one analysis over a nine-year period, the award-winning companies out-performed the S & P 500 share index by a ratio of almost 3:1. It prompted William Daley, the US Secretary of Commerce to comment "The fact is that quality pays. It pays in satisfied customers. It pays in motivated employees who are committed to their jobs. It pays in an improved bottom line."

The Cost of Quality

This term is widely misunderstood. The cost of quality is not the price of creating a quality product or service. It is the cost of *not* creating a quality product or service.

Philip Crosby, in *Quality is Free*, writes that the cost of quality is "the price of non-conformance" – in other words the cost of doing things wrong. This is often described by the term "cost of poor quality" (COPQ) because that implies what happens when continual improvement efforts are compromised.

Feigenbaum (see Chapter 2) believed that total quality control reduced operating costs stating that: "Quality and cost are complementary, not conflicting business objectives." He classified quality costs into three major cost categories:
• Prevention
• Appraisal
• Failure.

Prevention costs are incurred due to steps taken at the beginning of any process to protect against errors and defects and to incorporate quality into the service delivery process. They are incurred before services are provided and are therefore prospective and include costs associated with:
• Identification of clients' needs
• Education and training of employees
• Development of quality monitoring and reporting systems
• Institution of quality administration
• Management and planning.

Appraisal costs are related to appraising a service or products to ensure conformance to standards. They comprise the cost of resources that arise as a result of inspection activities, or in-practice preparation for the inspection, including audit.

Failure costs are divided into internal and external costs. Internal failure costs are those incurred as a result of redoing clinical work or avoidable remedial treatment; external failure costs relate to complaints, litigation, and the like.

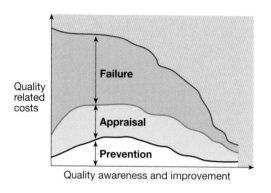

Fig 10-4 The relationship between quality related costs of prevention, appraisal and failure and increasing quality awareness and improvement within an organisation.

The relationship between quality related costs of these cost categories (known as the PAF model) and increasing quality awareness and improvement in the organisation are shown in Fig 10-4. The decreasing costs can be looked upon as a direct and tangible ROI.

Balanced Scorecard

The Balanced Scorecard is a conceptual framework for translating an organisation's vision and mission into a set of performance indicators. The concept was introduced by Professor Robert Kaplan and Dr David Norton in 1992, and has since been adopted by a wide range of organisations around the world. It is often quoted in the business press, having been the subject of a best-selling book in 1996.

Kaplan and Norton stress that no measure is sufficient by itself. They compare measuring performance along a single dimension with a pilot trying to fly an aeroplane by concentrating on airspeed alone and ignoring altitude. Failure to take a broadly-based view causes problems when implementing strategy, and they note that even the best-designed strategies often fail when it comes to implementation. People may fail to buy into the strategy as they feel their own aims are not represented.

Kaplan and Norton's model can yield the following benefits for the practice:
- Focusing the whole practice on the few key things needed to create breakthrough performance.
- Helping to integrate various practice initiatives, such as quality, re-engineering, and patient service improvements.
- Breaking down strategic measures so that team members can see how they can contribute to the overall business strategy.

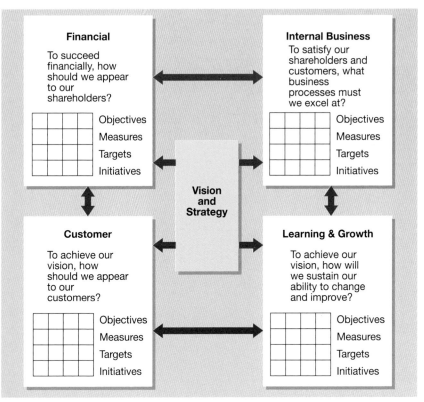

Fig 10-5 The Balanced Scorecard template. Adapted from Kaplan and Norton, 1996. The Balanced Scorecard. Harvard Business School Press: 9. Original from HBR Jan/Feb 1996, p. 76.

If used properly, the Balanced Scorecard becomes a catalyst for change. It is also a vehicle for implementing strategy and a tool for identifying pressure points, conflicting interests, objective setting, prioritisation, planning and budgeting (Fig 10-5). It offers managers a balanced view of their organisation upon which they can make strong decisions and upon which they can base real change. By using a Balanced Scorecard approach, we can rate overall performance by integrating financial measures with other key performance indicators. The four dimensions are:

- **Financial performance:** this measures the results the practice delivers to the stakeholders – profit for the owners and value for money where third party payments are concerned.

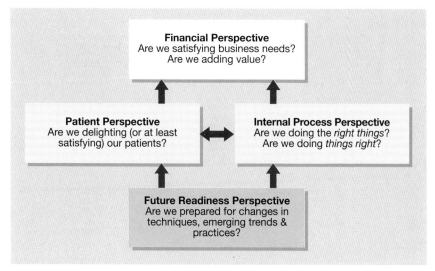

Fig 10-6 Questions to help complete the Balanced Scorecard.

- **Customer satisfaction:** this sees the practice through the eyes of the patients, measuring and reflecting on patient satisfaction.
- **Internal process improvement:** this focuses on the internal processes that drive the practice.
- **Learning and Growth:** this perspective is a measure of future performance based on the people and the infrastructure.

Adequate investment in these areas is critical to all long-term success and the questions we must ask are summarised in Fig 10-6.

Kaplan and Norton define their approach as follows: "The Balanced Scorecard translates an organisation's mission and strategy into a comprehensive set of performance measures that provide the framework for a strategic measurement and management system. The Balanced Scorecard retains an emphasis on achieving financial objectives, but also includes the performance drivers of those financial objectives. The scorecard measures organisational performance across four balanced perspectives: financial, customers, internal business processes, and learning and growth."

Summary

The unfortunate result of the quality revolution is that it is now offered or viewed as a strategic option that businesses should adopt. Quality management is an integral part of business management.

As we seek to define the meaning of quality, it is critical that we also understand that the objective of quality is customer satisfaction, and customer satisfaction is what businesses are about. If customer satisfaction is not the goal or the central focus, then the business has no business being in business.

"The ultimate quality award is improved bottom line profitability" was the opening statement of Bisgaard and Freiesleben's article about the economic case for quality in the September 2004 issue of Quality Progress, the journal of the American Society for Quality.

The authors went on to say that: "Satisfied customers come back for more and encourage business associates, family and friends to do the same." It reinforces a business maxim that was cited in the first in this series of books, namely that: "We do business with those we trust and we get business from those who trust us." That is quality realised.

Reference

Bisgaard S, Freiesleben J. Six Sigma and the Bottom Line. Qual Progress J 2004;37(9):57-62.

Index

Quintessentials for General Dental Practitioners Series

in 50 volumes

Editor-in-Chief: Professor Nairn H F Wilson

The Quintessentials for General Dental Practitioners Series covers basic principles and key issues in all aspects of modern dental medicine. Each book can be read as a stand-alone volume or in conjunction with other books in the series.

Publication date, approximately

Clinical Practice, Editor: Nairn Wilson

Culturally Sensitive Oral Healthcare	available
Dental Erosion	available
Special Care Dentistry	available
Evidence Based Dentistry	Spring 2007
Dental Bleaching	Spring 2007
Infection Control for the Dental Team	Spring 2007
Therapeutics and Medical Emergencies in the Everyday Clinical Practice of Dentistry	Summer 2007

Oral Surgery and Oral Medicine, Editor: John G Meechan

Practical Dental Local Anaesthesia	available
Practical Oral Medicine	available
Practical Conscious Sedation	available
Minor Oral Surgery in Dental Practice	available

Imaging, Editor: Keith Horner

Interpreting Dental Radiographs	available
Panoramic Radiology	available
Twenty-first Century Dental Imaging	Summer 2007

Periodontology, Editor: Iain L C Chapple

Understanding Periodontal Diseases: Assessment and Diagnostic Procedures in Practice	available
Decision-Making for the Periodontal Team	available
Successful Periodontal Therapy – A Non-Surgical Approach	available
Periodontal Management of Children, Adolescents and Young Adults	available
Periodontal Medicine: A Window on the Body	available

Endodontics, Editor: John M Whitworth

Rational Root Canal Treatment in Practice	available
Managing Endodontic Failure in Practice	available
Restoring Endodontically Treated Teeth	Spring 2007

Prosthodontics, Editor: P Finbarr Allen

Teeth for Life for Older Adults	available
Complete Dentures – from Planning to Problem Solving	available
Removable Partial Dentures	available
Fixed Prosthodontics in Dental Practice	available
Occlusion: A Theoretical and Team Approach	Spring 2007
Managing Orofacial Pain in Practice	Summer 2007

Operative Dentistry, Editor: Paul A Brunton

Decision-Making in Operative Dentistry	available
Aesthetic Dentistry	available
Communicating in Dental Practice	available
Indirect Restorations	available
Choosing and Using Dental Materials	Spring 2007
Composite Restorations in Posterior Teeth	Summer 2007

Paediatric Dentistry/Orthodontics, Editor: Marie Therese Hosey

Child Taming: How to Manage Children in Dental Practice	available
Paediatric Cariology	available
Treatment Planning for the Developing Dentition	available
Managing Dental Trauma in Practice	available

General Dentistry and Practice Management, Editor: Raj Rattan

The Business of Dentistry	available
Risk Management in General Dental Practice	available
Quality Matters: From Clinical Care to Customer Service	available
Practice Management for the Dental Team	Summer 2007

Dental Team, Editor: Mabel Slater

Team Players in Dentistry	Summer 2007

Implantology, Editor: Lloyd J Searson

Implantology in General Dental Practice	available

Quintessence Publishing Co. Ltd., London